Childhood Behaviour and Mental Health

Childhood behaviour and mental health

Michael Shepherd,
Bram Oppenheim
and Sheila Mitchell

University of London Press Ltd

ISBN 0 340 14769 5

University of London Press Ltd,
St Paul's House, Warwick Lane, London EC4P 4AH

Printed and bound in Great Britain by
W & J Mackay & Co Ltd,
Chatham, Kent

Contents

Acknowledgments

The authors would like to acknowledge the help of a number of people, without whose collaboration a study of this type could not have been undertaken. They are the Medical Director of St John's Hospital, Dr D. C. Watt, and the Management Committee of that hospital who provided local accommodation and working facilities; the former Medical Officer of Health of Buckinghamshire, Dr G. W. H. Townsend, the then Deputy Medical Officer of Health, Dr G. Knight, and the Director of Education, Mr R. Harding who furnished indispensable information; the consultants of the Child Guidance Clinics of the County, Dr C. E. Bagg, Dr E. Booth and Dr M. Pott who gave us access to their premises, records and patients; Dr D. C. Watt, Dr M. Heller, Dr R. R. Rodriguez, Dr P. A. Rogers and Mr J. Sant who undertook the arduous task of reading and rating the case-study profiles; and Miss Marjorie Cowell for help and advice in connection with the Hollerith analysis of the data. Finally, Mrs D. Plater, Mrs M. Bilsland, Miss J. Store and Miss I. McKnight provided invaluable assistance in typing and preparing the manuscript.

The work was supported by a grant from the Nuffield Provincial Hospitals Trust.

Figures

Tables

Chapter One

Introduction

'What is a child?' asked Bernard Shaw, and characteristically provided an answer: 'A fresh attempt to produce the just man made perfect: that is, to make humanity divine.' The language may be exaggerated, but the sentiments are so familiar and so consonant with modern thinking in the western world that we are apt to forget how recently they have become acceptable. Until the Renaissance the child took his place in society as a miniature adult, to be tolerated or exploited, treated with kindness or with cruelty as chance dictated, but always according to the standards of an adult world. In his survey of the changing role of children in family-life from the fifteenth century Philippe Ariès (1965) captures an era with one sentence: 'In medieval society the idea of childhood did not exist.'*

Modern concepts of childhood evolved gradually from the subsequent ferment in the history of European ideas. Undoubtedly the Christian gospel first exercised the principal influence in this sphere, as might have been expected when most teachers were members of the clergy with a vested interest in the future defenders of their faith. Individual thinkers of a less conformist nature and with a special bent towards education included men as diverse as Comenius, Locke, Rousseau and Herbart, but not until the nineteenth century was well advanced did the scientific approach to childhood begin to emerge as a field of investigation in its own right. Child study as we know it today originated in the thinking of the British evolutionary school (Keir 1952) and, in view of the contemporary climate of opinion, it did not go unopposed on either moral or social grounds. The theological basis of the anti-scientific, moralising argument is self-evident; even a progressive individual like Josephine Butler could write: 'It is a law of nature that children should suffer for the sins of their parents, and I do not think we can venture by legislative measures to interfere with that law.' Non-interference was also a convenient credo for the intensified exploitation of children which accompanied the industrial revolution. A

* All the references are given on p. 222ff.

number of well-entrenched social and political attitudes had to be eroded by enlightened legislation before it was possible to reach Trevelyan's verdict, that: 'As the nineteenth century grew older, humanity pervaded more and more all the dealings of life, particularly the treatment of children' (Trevelyan 1942).

With humanity came an awareness of the need for social action. At the same time as the industrial revolution was in full flow the introduction of universal education was bringing to light the importance of studying both normal and abnormal patterns of childhood behaviour. In Great Britain the Act of 1870 led to a sharp increase in the number of school attenders, with a consequent awareness of the surprisingly large number of seemingly ineducable children who were grouped together as 'mentally' or 'morally defective' and for whom further provision was required in the form of special schools and institutions. The size and nature of the problem exposed intensified the rising interest in child study as a scientific field of inquiry. In 1884 the genius of Francis Galton was responsible for the creation of an 'anthropometric laboratory' which included a scheme for the systematic investigation of individual children. Galton's ideas were elaborated and developed by Sully, who in 1893 established the British Child Study Association, primarily for psychologists and educationalists with an interest in this new discipline.

Even with the focus of attention on the individual child, however, it became quickly apparent that large-scale surveys were necessary for the purpose of both scientific inquiry and administrative action. Only in this way was it possible to provide reliable data about the characteristics of the child population at different phases of development and indicate the number of children likely to require special care. Binet's work in the field of psychometric testing demonstrated the value of this method in the cognitive sphere and Burt's early work for the London County Council was based on a clear definition of methods: 'First, an extensive survey has been made for general educational ability. This has embraced all the children upon the roll of ordinary and special (M.D.) schools, and has been based upon returns and estimates furnished by head teachers. Secondly, an intensive examination has been made of particular children and particular schools, including all the special (M.D.) schools, by the method of mental and scholastic tests. This has been done both to check the criteria employed by the teachers, and to examine the relation of proficiency in particular subjects to educational ability in general' (Burt 1917).

While these studies were understandably focused on measures of educational achievement they also served to direct attention to the importance of non-cognitive factors, not only by virtue of their influence on performance but also as phenomena in their own right (Burt 1935). The importance of emotional development was evident to the early child psychiatrists, but their outlook was generally confined by their concentration on individual clinical problems. The limitations of this viewpoint were recognised by Ackerson (1931, 1942) in his study of a consecutive series of 5 000 children examined at the Institute of Juvenile Research in Chicago between 1923 and 1927: from the records it was possible to obtain the distribution by age and sex of the incidence of 154 personality and conduct problems and to compute correlations between individual problems and other factors. Although Ackerson was aware of the bias in his sample of children he justified his procedure as unavoidable: 'Until parents can assume a more impersonal attitude towards the behaviour of their children and towards their own affairs, our only source of data for the scientific study of the more serious personality and conduct problems of children will be the somewhat selected group of children examined in behaviour or guidance clinics' (Ackerson 1931). Even at this time, however, it was possible to ask 'whether the children singled out for treatment are not, in an unduly high proportion, those who are a nuisance to parents or teachers rather than those making unsatisfactory social or personal adjustments' (McFie 1934) and to conclude that 'this obviously important question cannot be answered without discovering to what extent the different types of behaviour disorder and personality difficulty exists in our child population'.

Despite this admonition some years were to pass before the implications of this viewpoint, with its implicit call for what would now be termed epidemiological inquiry, were to be fully grasped by child psychiatrists (see page 156). However, as early as 1924 Wickman (1928), working as a psychologist at a demonstration child guidance clinic in the United States, attempted to determine the incidence of behaviour problems exhibited by children attending schools in Minneapolis and soon encountered a major difficulty. As a preliminary step all the teachers in a representative school were asked to list any form of behaviour which they regarded as constituting a 'problem': an analysis of the nature of the most frequently mentioned items revealed that they all involved behaviour which 'violates the teacher's principles of morality, her authority, the school or classroom order, the required standards of study, or disturbs through difficulties with other children'. Impressed by this bias, Wickman carried out a further investigation comparing the judgments recorded by teachers with those of specialists in mental hygiene. It then emerged that whereas the teachers had been principally concerned with outgoing, disruptive, anti-social conduct the mental hygienists had emphasised withdrawn behaviour as having more serious prognostic implications. Evidently the observers' preconceptions had influenced significantly their assessments, and these findings were confirmed by a number of investigators who conducted similar studies in the next two decades (Bain 1934, Ellis and Miller 1936, Goldfarb 1963, Hunter 1957, Laycock 1934, McClure 1929, Maes 1966, Mitchell 1942, Ritholz 1959, Schrupp and Gjerde 1953, Thompson 1940, Young-Masten 1938, Yourman 1932).

A recognition of this source of bias is apparent in the design of more sophisticated studies. Cummings (1944), for example, persuaded several teachers to keep a record of the behaviour of a random group of young children: Blatz and Bott (1927) had all the teachers in a school with 1400 pupils keep a twelve months' record of 'misdemeanours'; other workers have supplemented teachers' ratings with the impressions of other children from whom information was obtained by sociometric methods (Bower 1961, Mangus 1949, Ullman 1952). Individual items of behaviour have been studied with relative objectivity in classroom conditions: thus Olson (1929) has studied a series of 'nervous habits'—thumb-sucking, nail-biting hair-twiddling, nose-picking, ear-pulling, eye-rubbing—by observing and counting children's actions in class for twenty separate periods of five minutes, and direct inspection of the nails was employed in studies of nail-biting by Malone and Massler (1952) in the United States and by Birch (1955) in England.

Yet however comprehensive and carefully collected they may be data on school behaviour are always subject to one inescapable limitation: 'It must always be borne in mind that some children present a form of dual personality in respect to home and school. . . . Ascertainment of maladjusted children must include both teachers' and parents' viewpoints' (Schonell 1952). Though several studies have demonstrated how differently the same child may behave at home and at school (Eron *et al.* 1958, Pilzer 1952, Terman 1925), surprisingly few have explored the possibilities of using parental reports about the conduct of supposedly normal schoolchildren. For example, the pilot-study carried out in Birmingham for the Underwood Committee (1955) reported a 60–65 per cent agreement on psychologists' ratings of questionnaires by teachers and parents: of sixteen children in the survey who were seen subsequently by a psychiatrist at their parents' request, eleven had been rated free of maladjustment on the basis of their teachers' reports but, nevertheless, the other two pilot-studies carried out for this inquiry used the school reports as an initial screening device and parents were approached only when the teachers' assessment indicated some maladjustment on the part of the child.

Where information was obtained from parents, the difficulties involved in obtaining access to, and co-operation from, a representative sample has sometimes led to inquiries being confined to mothers from the higher socio-economic groups, with correspondingly higher educational standards (Goodenough 1931, Long 1941, Del Solar 1949). Griffiths (1952) made an attempt to survey childrens' behaviour by having questionnaires distributed to parents from sixteen schools, but unfortunately the principals concerned decided that they should determine the number of forms to be distributed in their own schools and presumably to the recipients, thus introducing a strong element of bias. More successful studies have been conducted by Mensh *et al.* (1959) and especially Lapouse and Monk (1958), whose aim was explicitly '. . . to penetrate the barriers of selection and to broaden knowledge about the behaviour, function and adjustment of children who are not likely to be picked out of the community for psychiatric examination and therefore have little chance of contributing to the statistics of symptoms'. For this purpose they administered a detailed interview schedule to several hundred mothers or mother-substitutes of children aged between six and twelve years, identified by interviewers who visited 1600 addresses systematically selected from a city directory.

As the range of cross-sectional studies extends to include observations at home, it might be anticipated that the recorded prevalence of deviant behaviour would increase. Since, however, such behaviour may represent no more than a temporary response to external factors, or even a phase of normal development rather than a disorder of mental health, any assessment of such conduct must take the duration into account. As Buckle and Lebovici (1960) have emphasised: 'All children show signs of disturbed behaviour at some time or another and professional intervention is justified only if the disorder persists long enough'. It is necessary in assessing the importance of any type of behaviour of children to use longitudinal studies to follow the natural history of the behaviour as well as cross-sectioned methods of measuring its prevalence at any point in time (Bell 1959–60, Moore 1965).

In general, longitudinal studies can be subdivided conveniently into those which are primarily concerned with the development of normal children and those which follow the progress of children with psychiatric disorders, usually to determine either the course of these conditions or the evaluation of their treatment. While the need to investigate children's emotional development is now widely acknowledged, the subject has been relatively neglected until recently for reasons which Chazan (1968) has summarised as follows '. . . the lack of measuring instruments, the failure to establish an acceptable theoretical framework within which research can be carried out, and the complexities of the study of emotional development, which is not easily amenable to laboratory experiment'. From Moore's review of the place of longitudinal research in the study of child development (Moore *et al.* 1954) it is apparent that the work on behaviour and personality is less clear-cut than that on physical and cognitive development.

The best-known early development studies were those of Gesell (1940, 1946, 1956), but the value of his detailed descriptions of normal behaviour was counterbalanced by the small size and highly selective nature of the sample, and the rather general nature of the information obtained from the mothers. Much of the early work was carried out in the United States and special mention must be made of the investigation by Macfarlane, Allen and Honzik (1954), who employed standardised recording forms and definitions of behaviour which were based on frequency and intensity so as to reproduce clear and systematic data about the distribution of various types of behaviour at different ages. More recently a longitudinal study of a group of socially homogeneous, middle-class New York Jewish children has provided data on the interaction between temperament and environment in the production of behaviour disorders (Chess, *et al.* 1963, Rutter *et al.* 1964, Chess *et al.* 1967), and at the Fels Institute several workers have attempted to relate children's conduct to the behaviour to their] parents (Baldwin *et al.* 1945, Baldwin 1947). In the United Kingdom three major longitudinal surveys of large representative groups of children have been undertaken. Two of them—Douglas' National Survey (Douglas 1964) and the 'Thousand Family' Survey in Newcastle upon Tyne (Spence *et al.* 1954, Miller *et al.* 1960)—were primarily oriented towards the physical health and illness of children born in the mid-1940s, though individual studies on mental health have been conducted in association with both surveys (Douglas and Mulligan 1961, Brandon 1960). The early results of the third study, under the auspices of the National Bureau for Co-operation in Child Care (Pringle *et al.* 1966) which involved 11 000 children born in the same week of March 1958, are only now becoming available. Another small British study of some 200 children in London has been concerned with a variety of emotional and personality characteristics, but few of the findings have been published so far (Moore *et al.* 1954, Moore 1959, Hindley 1965).

In contrast to the relative paucity of longitudinal studies designed to elucidate behavioural development there are numerous follow-up studies of children who have been referred to a treatment agency for one or other of the so-called behaviour disorders (Robins 1970). Some of these are simply descriptive reports on the condition of ex-patients after relatively short periods (Rexford and Schleifer 1956) or when they have entered adult life (Robinson 1951, Morris *et al.* 1954, O'Neal and Robins 1958a, 1958b). Other workers have analysed follow-up information in relation to a number of factors, including age (Wile *et al.* 1934), family characteristics (Barbour 1951, Cunningham *et al.* 1956, Wolff 1961), socio-economic status (Hubbard and Adams 1936), type of treatment (Witmer 1935) and clinical features (Cytryn *et al.* 1960, Rodrigues *et al.* 1959, Tyerman 1968). Such studies, however, have rarely compared the outcome of the treated groups with that of untreated children and, as a rule, favourable changes have been attributed to the treatment administered. Other work suggests that a more cautious interpretation is required. Thus Levitt (1957), on the basis of a review of published and unpublished data on treated children, concluded that approximately two-thirds recovered. He has also compared the results of treatment received by a group of children attending a child-guidance clinic with the fate of a group of 'defectors', i.e. children who were accepted for treatment at a diagnostic interview but then failed to attend for therapy. The two groups were similar in respect of clinical factors, social background, parental child-rearing practices and physical health and at follow-up five to six years later there was no apparent difference in outcome. These findings are in line with those reported by Powers and Witmer (1951) on the failure of 'counselling' to benefit a group of 325 'problem' children.

While the evidence from these studies suggests a trend towards the natural remission of many phenomena taken to indicate morbidity, it must be recalled that children who attend clinics cannot be regarded as representative of the whole universe of children with behavioural 'problems'. One of the few comprehensive attempts to study the persistence of such behaviour in 'normal' children was made by Macfarlane and her co-workers (1954), but the size of their sample had dwindled by the end of the follow-up period. With still smaller groups of young children Foster and Anderson (1930) and Cummings (1946), using parents' and teachers' reports respectively, found there to be a marked tendency for behavioural and emotional problems to disappear as the children grew older. On the basis of teachers' observations, other workers (Hildreth 1928, New York State Mental Health Research Unit 1964) have reported that only about one-third of the children exhibiting 'problems' on one occasion did so at a later date; unfortunately the informant was different on the two occasions, and it was not possible to determine whether the change represented a real improvement or a difference in the assessor's frame of reference.

It is evident from this brief review of a complex and scattered field that difficulties of both method and opportunity have combined to create a need for more information in several areas. Some of the more important of these can be summed up under four headings: (1) the nature and prevalence of many forms of behaviour believed to indicate emotional disorder; (2) the duration of such forms of behaviour; (3) the factors which distinguish 'problem' children who are referred to child-guidance clinics from other 'problem' children who are not so referred; (4) the degree to which 'improvement' in behaviour can be attributed to treatment rather than to development or environmental changes.

It was the objective of the set of investigations described in this volume to examine all four of these questions as a contribution to the study of mental health in childhood.

Chapter Two

Planning the survey of behaviour

Our first objective was to find out how behaviour problems were distributed in a population of supposedly 'normal' children. This immediately raised several practical questions: where to find a suitable population; how to obtain a sampling frame, and of what type; and how to gather the information required.

Selection of an area

There were two important considerations governing our choice of area. First, it had to be within a reasonable distance of the authors' place of work; secondly, it had to contain a reasonable cross-section of children living in varying types of social environment. The county of Buckinghamshire met both these criteria. In this county there are to be found rural areas, market towns and areas specialising in light industry; there are long-settled families, new London 'overspill' families and 'commuter-belt' families; and there are families of all social classes. It could therefore to some extent be regarded as representative of a wider area, the whole of southern England, though not necessarily of major urban areas, such as London, or of the heavy industrial areas in the north. An additional and important advantage lay in the interest and co-operation of the county health and education authorities.

Selection of information

From the outset we decided to obtain as comprehensive as possible a picture of the children's behaviour. Three possible informants were available—the parents, the teachers and the children themselves. A very strong theoretical case can be made out for using the child, who is most likely to have the fullest knowledge of how he feels and behaves at all times. There were, however, also a number of practical drawbacks to this procedure. First, it would not have been possible to use a comprehensive questionnaire because the younger children, and the less able of the older ones, would not have been sufficiently literate to complete it. To have circumvented this difficulty by interviewing the children individually would have involved more resources in the form of time, money and skilled personnel than were available to us unless we had severely limited the size of our sample. Interviewer-bias is also a major problem with children, and children attending the same school would certainly have discussed the questions among themselves. Also, Lapouse and Monk (1959) have suggested that children tend to be overscrupulous in reporting their own feelings and behaviour. They indicated, for example, that children might tell an interviewer that they had frightening dreams when there had been no evidence of this in their behaviour at the time and suggested that children, in an effort to be entirely truthful, may exaggerate their reports of their reactions to various situations. Finally, young children lack a frame of reference for questions dealing with frequency, e.g. 'often' or 'occasional'.

For these reasons we decided to use reports from the adults most closely concerned with the child—his parents, particularly his mother, and his teachers. Both approaches were thought necessary since there seemed no certainty that a child's behaviour at school would necessarily correspond with his behaviour at home (von Harnack 1953, 1958). We placed the main emphasis, however, on the mother's* description, since a mother has most opportunity to develop an intimate and comprehensive knowledge of many aspects of her child's behaviour, e.g. eating, sleeping, waking, sick or well.

It might be argued that a mother's descriptions can provide only one individual's way of perceiving the child's behaviour: the way in which she records the behaviour will depend on her expectations as well as on the child's conduct. Her assessment of the child's appetite, for instance, will depend on what she considers to be the normal consumption of food by a child of that age and sex. Standards may vary considerably, but if any mother considers that her child's behaviour is in some way aberrant, this belief will affect the way in which she perceives the child and reacts to

* 'Mother' is practically synonymous with 'parent' in this case, as the results of the survey showed that in most cases questionnaires were completed by mothers (or mother-substitutes) alone, about 10 per cent by mother and father in combination, and only very few by fathers alone.

him. In the context of this study, mother and child have perforce to be regarded as a dual entity whose 'problem' may consist either of the child behaving in a way that is deviant or of the mother's perception of his behaviour as deviant. In studies of this type, as Pringle *et al.* (1966) have pointed out, 'one is essentially obtaining a measure of a relationship between two persons'.

The parents' questionnaire

After reviewing the range of available questionnaires we decided that the one constructed by Cattell and Coan (1957) would provide a useful basis for our own study. In its original form this consisted of fifty-three sets of three statements, covering a broad range of behaviour and personality traits; in each set, the mother was asked to underline the statement which best applied to her own child, e.g. 'rarely cries—cries about as much as most children of the same age—cries more than most children'. Using this questionnaire in its original form, we carried out pilot interviews with twenty mothers, chiefly recruited through preliminary visits to schools in various parts of Buckinghamshire. In each case the head teacher was asked to suggest names of people who would be representative of the mothers of pupils at his school. At the interview the mother was asked to complete the questionnaire, thinking aloud as she did so and making any comments or mentioning any doubts that occurred to her. The interviewer (S.M.) stressed that we were trying to find questions which would be clear to everybody, and that we wanted to know whether any question seemed confusing or difficult to understand.

The comments noted during these interviews made it obvious that in its original American form some items of the questionnaire were misleading to a Buckinghamshire respondent: for instance, 'rarely complains' was taken to mean 'rarely suffers from ailments' by several mothers. Taking these comments into account we prepared an amended draft of the questionnaire and interviewed a second group of others. Again, we found several ambiguous questions, so that further reorganisation of the questions and their wording was undertaken.

In addition, two more fundamental difficulties emerged at this phase of the inquiry. First, it became obvious that the questions covered two different aspects of behaviour. Some dealt with *intensity* of behaviour, e.g. 'dislikes going to school—likes school about as much as most children—likes school very much'; others dealt with *frequency* of behaviour, e.g. 'no bed-wetting—occasional bed-wetting—frequent bed-wetting'. In both cases, the mother had to use her own frames of reference in deciding whether to reply, for example, that her child disliked school more than 'most children' or that the child's weekly headaches were 'occasional' or 'frequent'? It seemed evident that we could only obtain a clearer picture of the true state of affairs by a more rigorous definition of our categories, particularly in respect of frequency.

A pilot study was therefore carried out in London. Mothers were interviewed and asked to explain in more detail what they meant by the general description, e.g. 'occasional', 'frequent', which they applied to their child's behaviour. The need for some clarification of terms soon became apparent: 'occasional tummy pains', for instance, ranged in frequency from almost daily to no more than once a year. To avoid this confusion we decided to phrase questions dealing with frequency in terms of an eight-point scale, as follows: *a*) every day or almost every day; *b*) two or three times a week; *c*) about once a week; *d*) about once every two weeks; *e*) about once a month; *f*) about once in two or three months; *g*) two or three times a year; *h*) never or less than once a year.

It was also necessary to consider whether the behaviour items included in the questionnaire were all relevant to our purpose and whether the selection of items covered was sufficiently comprehensive. Some of the original items dealt solely with personality or character, e.g. 'talks in rather a quiet voice—speaks in about as loud a voice as most children—talks in rather a loud voice'. Such statements have little clinical significance and are difficult to evaluate. On the other hand, some common forms of behaviour often regarded as psychiatric 'problems' (Kanner 1962) had been omitted from the original questionnaire, e.g. tics, withdrawn behaviour, wandering, truancy and mood swings. Items were therefore designed to include some of these phenomena. We did not include grossly delinquent acts, such as arson or assault, overtly obsessional or bizarre behaviour or abnormal sexual activities, since the inclusion of such items might well have upset some parents and so have reduced our response rate without providing us with any additional information. Cases of major psychiatric disorder or delinquency would be rare in a sample of children attending normal schools and in any case their presence would be strongly indicated by the mother's responses to the other items which were already included in the questionnaire.

In addition to the main section on behaviour, the parents' questionnaire (see Appendix 3) also asked for information on two aspects of the child's life with obvious relevance to his psychological state. First, there was a set of questions about physical health and medical history in terms of symptoms, illness and admission to hospital. Secondly, several items bearing on the social and personal history were included, e.g. family position, separation from parents, family disruption, whether or not the mother worked, the social status of the family and the length of time the family had lived in the community.

As the information sought from parents was personal, no name or address appeared on the questionnaires, which were identified by serial numbers. This ensured that the information was kept confidential.

The questionnaire as a discriminating instrument

Once the questionnaire had been provisionally drafted, our next step was to examine how far it distinguished between those children with and without known behaviour disorders. For this purpose another pilot study was carried out.

The names of forty-eight children of school age were taken consecutively from the waiting lists of the three child guidance clinics in the country. These children had been referred for psychiatric advice and therefore might reasonably be supposed to be showing some evidence of disordered behaviour. Each child was matched by age and sex with another child selected by his teacher as exemplifying well-adjusted behaviour. For all children in both groups, a questionnaire was sent to the mother by post with a covering letter and a stamped, addressed envelope for the return of the completed form. About a week later, a reminder was sent to the mothers who had not returned their questionnaires. In two areas mothers who still failed to reply were then visited to determine whether their refusal was related to adverse feeling towards any particular item in the questionnaire; this did not appear to be the case. In all, ninety-two questionnaires were returned out of ninety-six. In each case a crude score was calculated by allocating one point for each item where the behaviour was reported to occur at the most extreme intensity or at an arbitrary frequency of more than once a month.* The results are set out here in table 1.

* A more refined method, based on the statistical probability of the behaviour occurring at any age in each sex was used for the analysis of data in the main survey (see pages 76–8).

TABLE I. *Cumulative percentage of children showing the number of extreme items on questionnaires*

Number of extreme items marked	*Parents' forms*		*Teachers' forms*	
	Clinic children cum. %	*Non-Clinic children cum. %*	*Clinic children cum. %*	*Non-Clinic children cum. %*
More than 12	8·3	Nil	Nil	Nil
" " 10	16·7	Nil	Nil	Nil
" " 8	19·4	Nil	Nil	Nil
" " 6	44·4	Nil	8·3	Nil
" " 4	52·8	2·8	30·6	Nil
" " 2	83·3	22·2	50·0	Nil
At least 1	97·2	66·7	97·2	19·4

From these figures it appeared that the questionnaire was successful in distinguishing between the two groups. The information cannot, of course, be taken to validate the form as a diagnostic instrument; it did, however, suggest that the questionnaire could usefully collect data on items of behaviour which were prevalent among children referred to child guidance clinics. The degree of discrimination between individual items varied. Behaviour which interfered with social relations appeared to separate the groups widely: such conduct included irritability, temper tantrums, restlessness, disobedience, mood swings, lying, food fads, reading difficulties and worry. Most of the other items, however, also revealed differences between groups, although these were less substantial.

The teachers' questionnaire

In planning the teachers' questionnaire we had to balance two different requirements: first, the need for as much information as possible about each child in his school environment and, secondly, our recognition that other calls on the teachers' time must necessarily limit the amount of detailed information they could be expected to supply. We first prepared a questionnaire and asked the head teachers of twenty schools of all types whether their staff could reasonably be expected to provide answers to our questions. This resulted in a number of valuable suggestions and an amended version of the form was prepared for use in a pilot investigation of forty-eight matched pairs of children.

In general, the questions asked of the teachers were designed to cover two broad areas of the children's conduct: academic performance and problems of health and behaviour.

ACADEMIC PERFORMANCE

The schools in Buckinghamshire varied widely in nature, size, organisation, curriculum and type of pupil. There were small village primary schools with only two classes, infants and juniors, to cover all ages from five to eleven; there were large urban schools in which a one-year intake of children might be divided into four or more streams, each consisting of thirty-five to forty children. After eleven years of age, the system was, at the time of the investigation, selective, with children attending grammar, technical or secondary modern schools according to their performance in the eleven-plus tests and to parental preference. In considering academic performance we could have made an overall comparison using the eleven-plus arithmetic and English texts for the older children. We decided, however, that such an exercise would add little of value to our study, for, apart from broad categories, which were already known to us through the selection procedure and merit streaming within schools, a child's attainment in terms of two basic standardised tests at ten or eleven years of age did not seem to offer much help in assessing actual performance within a particular school environment in later years. We could also have used some of the standardised group tests available to obtain for each child an estimate of IQ and of attainment in some individual subjects. However, it was decided that in view of the aims of our study, such a procedure would be uneconomical. For our purposes the important factor was the child's position within his own age group in his own school and particularly within his own classroom. We therefore adopted the very simple but eminently feasible procedure of asking teachers to assess whether the child's usual position in class was in the top 25 per cent, the bottom 25 per cent or the middle 50 per cent; we asked for an assessment of attainment in general and of reading ability relative to children of the same age attending the same type of school. We also obtained information about the streaming system used in the school and the relative position of the child's class within that system. From this basic information it was possible to classify each child in terms of academic attainment in his own particular school setting.

HEALTH AND BEHAVIOUR

The types of behaviour on which teachers were asked to report were limited to those which could, under normal circumstances, be observed by them in the school environment. We did not, for instance, ask them about bed-wetting or food fads. The items included in the teachers' form approximated, in most instances, to the types of behaviour covered by the parents' questionnaire, but for the teachers we did not offer a multiple choice of intensity or frequency for each type of behaviour. We merely asked them to indicate whether the problem described applied to the child being considered. Information about medical disability was sought in an open-ended question and space was left for the comments of those teachers, usually in infant or junior schools, who felt that they would like to give a more detailed and personal account of the child.

Approaching the parents

The next problem was to determine the method of approach to parents which would result in the greatest number of questionnaires being completed and returned. Three methods were tried.

1. A random sample of 100 children was chosen from the school medical cards for one area of Buckinghamshire. In each case a questionnaire was sent direct by post to the mother, who was asked to complete and return it in the stamped, addressed envelope provided.

2. A further random sample of 100 children was taken from the same school medical record cards, but this time the questionnaires were sent to the children's mothers through the schools concerned. In each case the head teacher was asked to give to the child a sealed envelope addressed to the mother and containing a questionnaire, a covering letter and an envelope addressed to the research team. After completing the form the parents had simply to seal it into the envelope which the child then brought back to school and gave to his teacher. The forms for each school were collected together and returned to the team unopened. In the letter to the parents it was stressed that the teacher would *not* open the envelopes or read what the parents had written. This was also stressed in the letter sent to the head teachers taking part in the project.

3. A whole class of children was chosen from each of four schools randomly selected from a stratified list of all local authority schools in the county, and every child in the sample class was given a questionnaire to take home. The subsequent procedure then followed the same pattern as that of the second method. The four schools selected were *a*) a mixed

grammar school in a fairly new urban area with some L.C.C. overspill; *b*) a village primary school with only two classes, one for infants aged five to seven years and one for juniors of seven to eleven; *c*) a mixed primary school in a small town; and *d*) a mixed secondary modern school in a predominantly rural area. The class to be used was, in each case, chosen after discussion with the head teacher. In two of the schools the research worker was asked to explain to the children the purpose of the survey and why they had been chosen to help. In the other two schools this was done by the headmaster.

TABLE 2. *Response rates by three methods of approach to parents*

	Number of questionnaires	Number of questionnaires never received by parents because of removal etc.	Number of questionnaires completed	Number of questionnaires received but not completed by parents
Sent by post direct to parents	100	11	55	34
Sent to sample parents via school	100	6*	85†	9
Sent to parents via school (whole class)	137	Nil	131 (96%)	6

* *Including two cases where the form was not sent to parents by the school because of parental illness.*
† *This includes three children who had changed school but whose forms were forwarded by the old school.*

Table 2 shows the response rates obtained by the three methods. It can be clearly seen from this table that the transmission of the parents' questionnaires by the school was much more successful than a direct approach through the post. Of the two methods involving the school, that which used the whole class was found to be somewhat more successful than the one based on a random sample of children, partly because there was less waste through failure to make contact with the parents. When a whole class was used we obtained the names from the school register, prepared the forms at the school and gave them to the children on the same day, so that we could be sure that no one had left the area. On the other hand, this method of approach made it virtually impossible to use the teachers' questionnaire, since no teacher could in charity be asked to complete forty forms. As a result, it was decided that we should adopt the second method for the main project, i.e. obtain a sample of children through the school health record cards and send the questionnaires to parents through the children's schools. Provided that errors were eliminated, we could expect a response rate from the parents of about 90 per cent and a teacher's report for every child.

Chapter Three

The survey of behaviour: sampling and field work

The main sample

In April 1961 we started to draw the sample for the main survey. Relatively large numbers were desirable to ensure coverage of infrequent items of behaviour: the method consisted in picking out every tenth card from the school medical record cards which were filed in the offices of each of the seven divisional health areas of the county. It was, however, by no means certain that the sample children would be available to receive their questionnaires at the school recorded on their health cards. These tended in some areas to reflect the situation at the child's last school medical examination. In several cases the records had not been amended when children moved from primary to secondary school, when they transferred to private schools, when they moved from one area of the town or county to another, or when they left the county altogether.

As a precaution, we prepared a list of children believed to be attending each school and asked each head teacher to check whether this was the case. To make up for any deficiences, reserves were obtained by picking a second sample of 1 in 140 and these were also included in the lists sent to the schools. When the lists were returned, children who had changed schools within the county were traced to their new school when possible. Any child who had left the county or disappeared entirely was replaced by a reserve.

Supplementary sampling

NEW SCHOOL ENTRANTS

When the main sample was drawn we could not include most of the five-year-old children who had started school during the 1960–1 school year, since most of them were not given their first school medical examination until later in the year and so had no medical cards. As this age group is of special importance we drew a further 1 in 10 sample from these children's cards as soon as they were made out.

SPECIAL SCHOOLS

At the time of the main survey we did not include any children who were at special schools. These children comprised three groups: *a*) children who could not cope with an ordinary school course because they suffered from a major physical defect, e.g. children who were blind, deaf or spastic; *b*) children who could not cope with an ordinary school course because of intellectual or emotional difficulties, e.g. educationally subnormal children, maladjusted children; *c*) children who probably could have coped with a normal school course, but who had been sent to special schools in the belief that a change of environment would benefit their physical or mental health, e.g. 'delicate' children, asthmatics and some maladjusted children.

No study of children's behaviour could be comprehensive if it did not cover at least the two later groups. It was, therefore, decided that a 1 in 10 sample should be selected from all the children whose homes were in Buckinghamshire and who had been placed in special schools either inside or outside the county by the county education authority.

CHILDREN ATTENDING PRIVATE SCHOOLS

Much attention was given to the possibility of improving the representativeness of our sample by including pupils in fee-paying schools. Unfortunately, however, this procedure did not appear feasible. For instance, as there was no central register from which a sample of names could be drawn, it would have been necessary to obtain a list of pupils' names and addresses from each of the 101 fee-paying schools in the county not all of which might have wished to co-operate. Moreover, even if this task had been possible, many of the larger schools drew their pupils from outside Buckinghamshire, and, conversely, Buckinghamshire children might well be at boarding schools in other parts of the country. We felt, however, that we should be able to estimate the extent of the gap which existed in our coverage. Consequently, a letter was sent to the principal of each independent school in the county asking for information about the number of pupils of appropriate age who came from homes within the county.

Replies were received from eighty-eight of the schools approached.

After estimates were made for the other thirteen it was found that approximately six thousand children of between five and fifteen who were at private schools had been omitted from our study. This has resulted in an under-representation of children from Social Classes I and II.

Despatch of questionnaires

After the lists had been checked, we were left with a sample of 6463 children from 330 schools. Every school* received a set of envelopes each addressed by name to a particular mother, a list of the children in the sample and a covering letter to the head teacher. In addition, there was a teacher's report form for every child on the list. The head teachers, who by now were fully aware of the survey procedure, were asked to hand the envelopes to the children concerned and to ask class teachers to complete a teacher's form for each of these children. Inside each envelope was an explanatory letter addressed to the mother, a questionnaire and an addressed envelope for its return. The teachers were asked to collect the completed questionnaires from the children and to forward them, unopened, to us.

As the lists for the schools had already been checked, the loss through removal was trivial, though a small number of children had moved since the lists were checked and some errors had occurred in the checking. However, over the whole county only sixty-seven children (1·0 per cent) could not be reached. A further small loss of thirty-nine children occurred because three schools decided that they could not take part.

Questionnaire returns

For the sample as a whole, 93 per cent of the questionnaires received by parents were returned fully or mostly completed. For the teachers, the equivalent return rate was 97 per cent. There were only small differences in the return rates from different parts of the county.

Since the teachers' questionnaires were available for most of the children whose parents had failed to return the questionnaire, it was possible to obtain some data on which to compare the children whose parents had responded and those whose parents had not. The two groups

* This procedure did not apply to residential special schools: questionnaires were posted direct to the parents of children attending such schools, not sent through the school.

differed in several important characteristics.* The children of non-responding parents were more likely to be boys and, in particular, boys over the age of eleven. For each sex, the children of non-responders were much more likely to be graded by their teachers as below average in attainment: 53 per cent of boys and 40 per cent of girls compared with 34 per cent and 24 per cent respectively among children whose parents completed questionnaires. With regard to behaviour in school, boys whose parents had not completed questionnaires were more likely than the other boys to be described as 'uninterested in school work' (18 per cent of non-responders: 6 per cent of responders), 'unco-operative in class' (10 per cent: 4 per cent), 'often tells lies' (9 per cent: 3 per cent), and 'has stolen things on one or more occasions' (5 per cent: 2 per cent). Among the girls, on the other hand, the only recorded differences between the behaviour in school of children of responders and non-responders were that the latter were more likely to be rated 'unco-operative in class' (5 per cent: 2 per cent) and to have 'stolen things on one or more occasions' (4 per cent: 1 per cent). For both sexes, children whose forms were not returned were more likely to be absent from school 'for odd days and half-days for no good reason but apparently with the support and knowledge of their parents'.

From these results, it appears likely that the omission from our survey of the children whose parents did not complete forms may have led to an underestimation of the number of children with behaviour problems in the school population. This is particularly true of the male population, and it seems probable that some boys with delinquent tendencies were omitted from our survey.†

* The differences outlined in this section were all statistically significant at a 1 per cent level using a chi-square test.

† This is supported by a follow-up study (Taylor, 1968) which showed that a higher than expected proportion of children whose parents did not complete forms had appeared in court since the survey.

Chapter Four

The child at home

The survey described in Chapter 3 provided us with information about more than six thousand schoolchildren, forming a fairly representative cross-section of all the children at local authority schools in Buckinghamshire (tables 3 and 4). From the data supplied by the parents it was possible

TABLE 3. *Distribution of sample schoolchildren by age and sex*

Age at last birthday		*Boys*	*Girls*
5 years		251	209
6		356	312
7		369	336
8		342	336
9		319	291
10		308	289
11		315	314
12		307	270
13		321	292
14		322	336
15		44	56
Not recorded		4	5
	Total	3258	3046

TABLE 4. *Distribution of sample schoolchildren by age, sex and father's occupation*

Father's occupation	*Boys* aged 5–10 years	*Boys* aged 11–15 years	*Girls* aged 5–10 years	*Girls* aged 11–15 years
Professional, administrative, managerial, executive and supervisory (higher grade)	425	222	392	256
Supervisory (lower grade) and other non-manual	306	163	247	186
Skilled manual	685	427	591	440
Semi-skilled and routine manual	531	339	465	304
Unemployed and disabled	3	3	5	8
Not recorded	69	85	73	79
Totals	2 019	1 239	1 773	1 273

to obtain a picture of the comparative distribution of each type of behaviour in children of each sex at any age from five to fifteen.

Analysis of types of behaviour

In this chapter each type of behaviour is analysed separately though, for convenience, we have grouped items together under a number of broad headings. The wording of the items can be seen on the figures and, in addition, the item number on the appropriate questionnaire (see Appendix 3, page 212) has been entered in brackets after the appropriate sub-heading.*

FEEDING BEHAVIOUR

Appetite (Q.55)

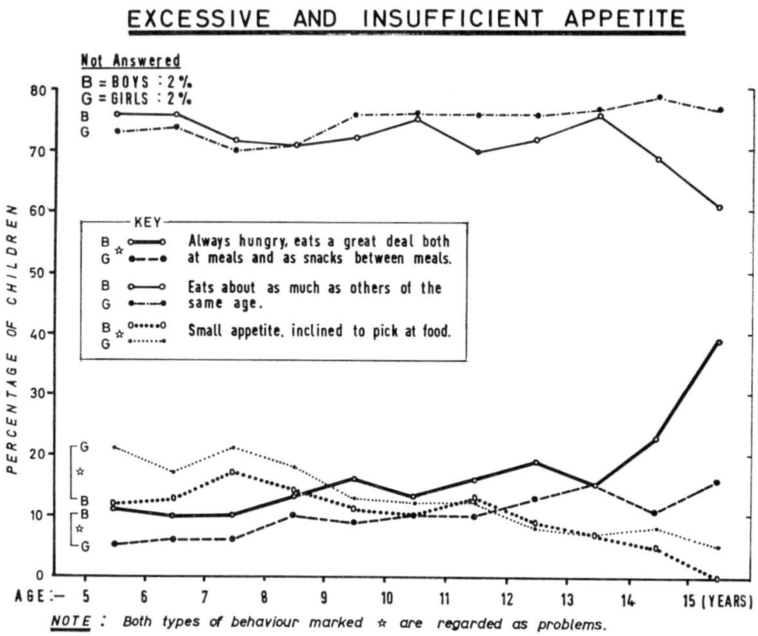

FIGURE I

The distribution of intensity of appetite may be taken as indicating 'problem' behaviour at both extremes of the scale: at one end is the child with

* Probabilities where quoted refer to testing significance by means of a chi-square test using Yates' correction where appropriate.

an excessively large appetite, at the other the child who eats very little and picks at his food.

a. *Large appetite* The prevalence of large appetites was found to increase with age, reaching its peak in both sexes at fifteen years. At almost every age, boys were more likely than girls to be considered 'always hungry'. This difference was particularly marked at the age of fifteen years, when 39 per cent of the boys were said to have insatiable appetites compared with 16 per cent of the girls ($P < 0·05$).

b. *Small appetite* The high prevalence of parent's complaints about poor appetite has been noted by many clinicians. Mackenzie (1953), for instance, suggests that at least one such case is seen weekly in paediatric practice, and Kanner (1957) talks of it as 'a widespread cultural phenomenon in our midst'. In the present study one child in every eight (12·5 per cent) was reported as having a small appetite. The prevalence rate, however, varied with age (see figure 1). Thus, among the five- to ten-year-olds 17 per cent of girls and 13 per cent of boys were classified as poor eaters compared with 9 per cent of girls and 8 per cent of boys among those of eleven or older ($P < 0·001$ in each case). It is also noteworthy that, in the younger age group, girls were more likely than boys to be described as having small appetites ($P < 0·001$); this was not true of the older children between the ages of eleven and thirteen years, among whom the picture was reversed.

Macfarlane *et al.* (1954) found no difference in the prevalence rates of boys and girls but did note a tendency for the problem to decrease in frequency as the children became older.

Food fads (Q.53)

Although between 40 and 50 per cent of all the children in the survey were said to 'eat nearly anything', fussiness about food was nevertheless reported of about one in five boys up to the age of eleven years and the same proportion of girls up to the age of ten years. Among still older children the frequency decreased slightly, but food fads were still recorded for at least one in seven of the older children. The peak age was eleven for boys and ten for girls though, on the whole, the age-curve can be seen to be relatively flat. The distribution of food fads in the population was slightly higher among boys than among girls at most ages. The difference, however, was significant only among the eleven-year-olds ($P < ·05$).

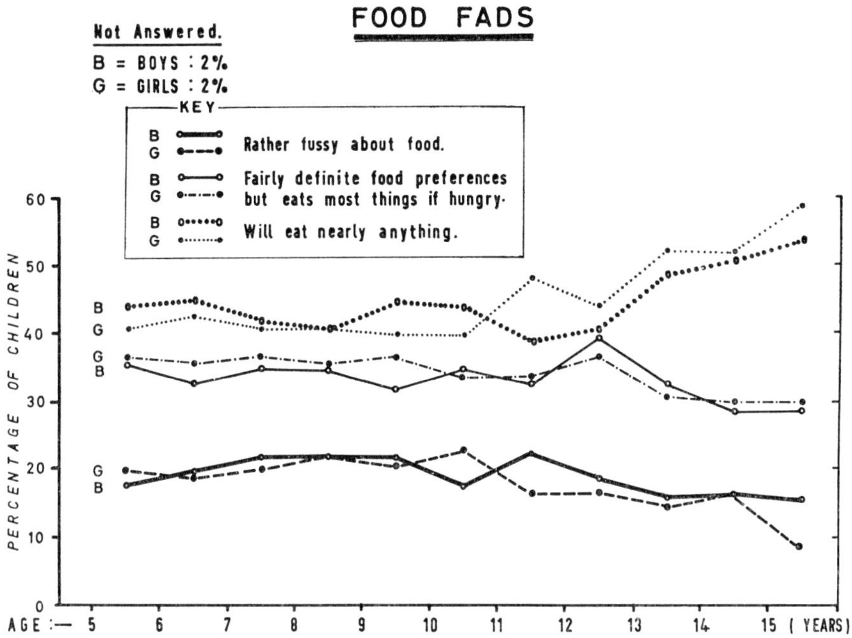

FIGURE 2

Previous studies have varied in approach and coverage, and their diversity is apparent from the reported findings. Baldwin (1944), an expert on nutrition, interviewed seventy-six mothers as part of the Fels Institute research project and found that 56 per cent of the children investigated were 'unreasonably finical'. Ackerson (1931) found 'finicky food habits, capricious appetite' among 8 per cent of the girls and 10 per cent of the boys attending clinics. He found that there was little variation in frequency with age among boys but that the prevalence among girls was reduced after the age of twelve. Gesell and Ilg (1946) say that 'preferences and refusals become less marked after the age of eight years'. Their data, however, were derived from the examination of about fifty American children who were of high socio-economic class and above average intelligence. Macfarlane *et al.* (1954) found a peak of food faddiness at the age of six, when 29 per cent of boys and 51 per cent of girls were included in this category; the frequency then fell sharply to only 4 per cent of boys and 9 per cent of ten-year-old girls, although there was again an increase at the age of twelve to 17 per cent and 24 per cent respectively.

FEARS

Four types of fear were included in the parents' questionnaire—fear of the dark, fear of animals, fear of strangers and extreme shyness or fear of other children. The data for each type of behaviour are discussed separately below. If, however, we consider the total group of fears covered, it is apparent that the distributions are of two types. On the one hand, reactions to animals and the dark were clearly related to age: among the five-year-olds about half of the sample showed some degree of uneasiness in each of these two fields, but this proportion rapidly diminished as the children became older. In the other group of fears—of strange adults and strange children—there was very little association with age. It would seem reasonable to suggest that shyness, at least to some degree, is a facet of the child's personality rather than a transient phase of development; it can also be seen from figures 5 and 6 that children are less likely to feel shyness in the company of other children than when they are among strange adults.

Fear of the dark (Q.48)

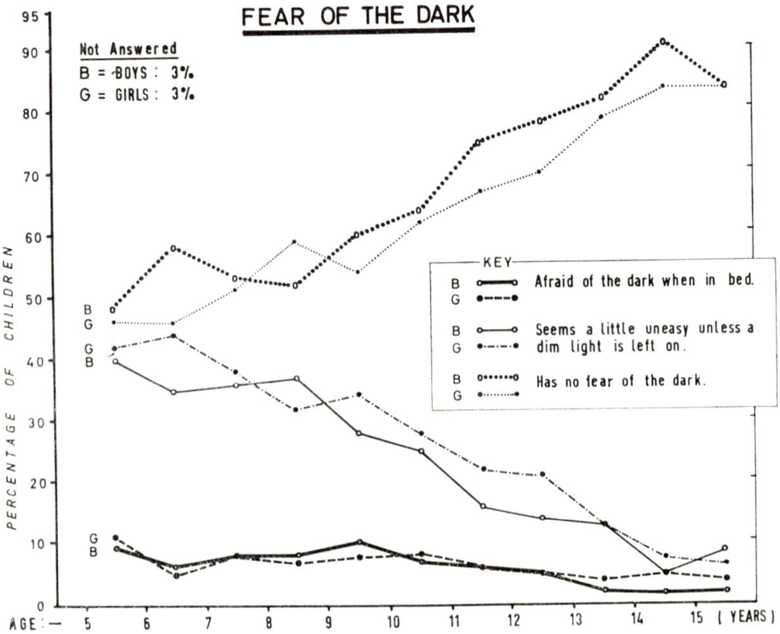

FIGURE 3

Fear of the dark when in bed at night was the most commonly occurring fear in both sexes at all ages. In each sex, the proportion of children said to be afraid of the dark remained relatively constant up to the age of ten and then declined. The milder category of 'uneasiness' unless a light was left on, however, showed a regular fall with increasing age; conversely, the proportion of children showing no fear rose from less than half of the five-year-olds to about 60 per cent at eleven years of age and more than 80 per cent of those aged fourteen and fifteen. Lapouse and Monk (1959) reported such fears to be more common among six- to eight-year-olds than among those aged nine to twelve.

As can be seen from figure 3, there was very little difference in the proportion of girls and boys who were afraid of the dark at any age up to thirteen. However, girls were, on the whole, more likely than boys to be uneasy in the absence of a light.

Fear of animals (Q.46)

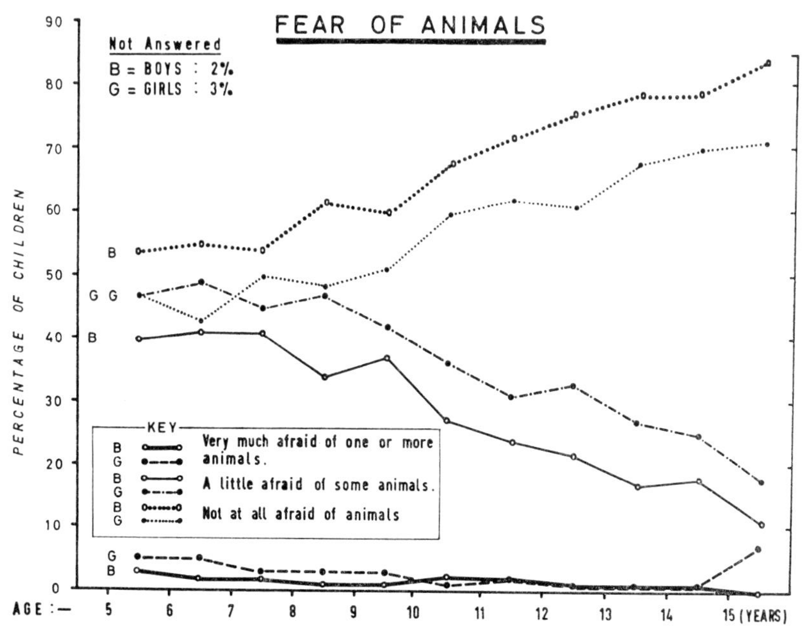

FIGURE 4

It is apparent from figure 4 that while only a small minority of school children showed great fear of animals, at least one-third of those under eleven were described as being 'a little afraid'. It is also clear that such fear was most frequently reported in the younger age-groups and decreased steadily with age. Similar findings have been noted by Lapouse and Monk (1959), Cummings (1944) and Jersild and Holmes (1935). It is probable that the peak incidence occurs in the pre-school period: Macfarlane *et al.* (1954) found fear of dogs most marked among three-year-olds.

At all ages, girls were more likely than boys to be described as showing slight fear of some animals. Among those who showed extreme fear there was a sex difference up to the age of nine years, when the prevalence rate for girls (4 per cent) was twice as great as for boys (2 per cent) ($P < 0{\cdot}01$). The sex difference appeared again at fifteen years, when 7 per cent of the girls, but none of the boys, were said to be very frightened of some animal. This difference may indicate that girls are particularly likely to experience such fears in adolescence, but the number of fifteen-year-olds included in the survey was small (fifty-six girls, forty-four boys) as we included only those of the statutory school age. It could be, therefore, that a few atypical cases carried undue weight.

Fear of meeting people (Q.47)

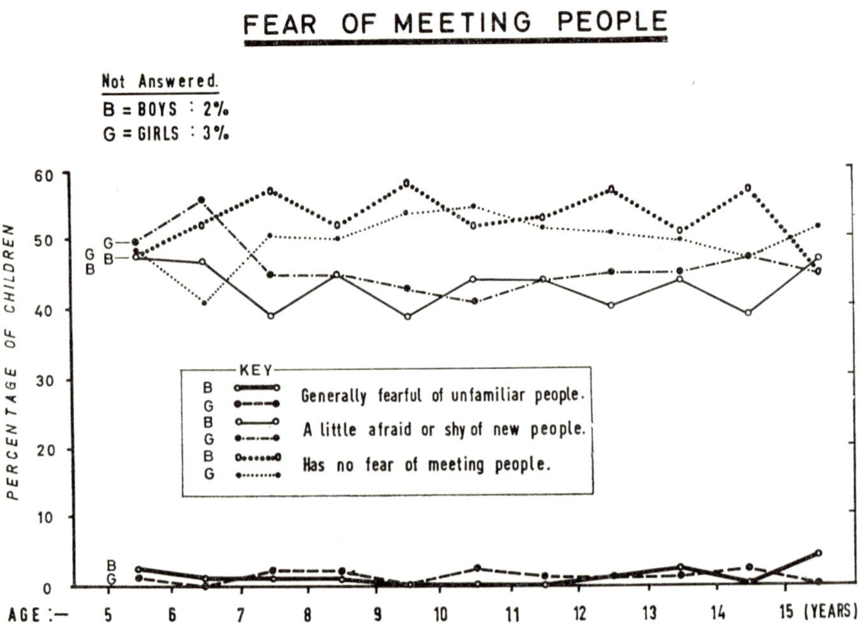

FIGURE 5

Figure 5 shows that the most extreme category on this item, i.e. 'generally fearful of unfamiliar people' was rarely underlined. Indeed, it was only applied to thirty-seven girls (12 per thousand) and twenty-eight boys (9 per thousand) out of the whole sample. 'A little' fear or shyness of new people was, however, relatively common, being reported of nearly half the children in the sample. By contrast to the two types of fear already discussed, this shyness did not bear any consistent relation to age. Thus, the proportion of shy boys fluctuated between 39 and 45 per cent with a slight rise in the youngest and oldest age group; the curve for girls had its peak among the five- to six-year-olds, fell to its lowest point at ten years and rose again with the approach of adolescence.

In the extreme category, there was no relation between fear of unfamiliar people and the child's sex, but at most ages girls were a little more likely to show some signs of shyness than were boys.

Shyness of other children (Q.54)

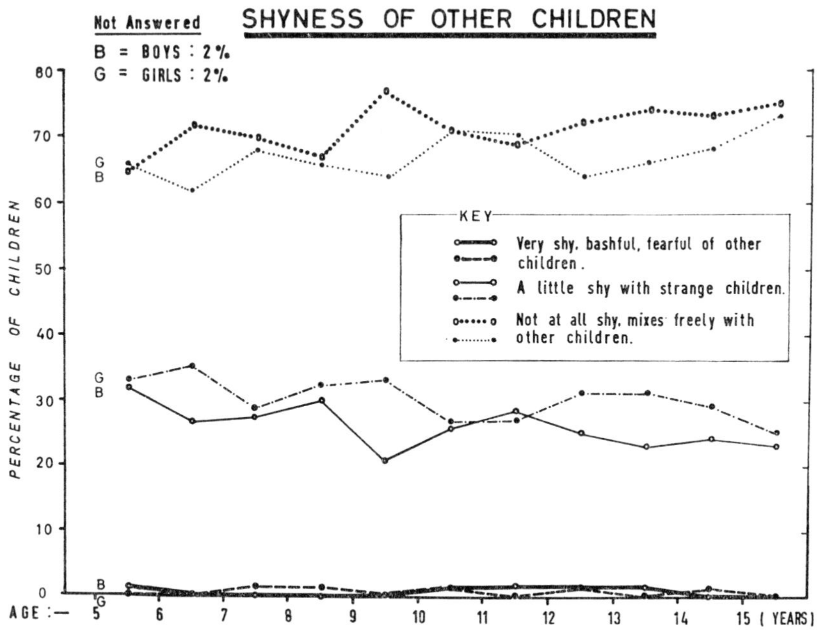

FIGURE 6

This item was the least common of the fears, being reported at extreme intensity of only nineteen girls (6 per thousand) and seventeen boys (5 per thousand) studied. These figures show no sex differences but an analysis of the data by age (see figure 6) indicates that the boys tended to develop such feelings only after the age of nine years, whereas the girls showed a fairly regular picture at all ages.

In the moderate category the picture was very similar to generalised shyness towards new people which has already been discussed: the curve remained relatively constant at all ages, and girls were a little more likely to show some shyness towards strange children than were boys. The proportion of children feeling shy with their own contemporaries was, however, smaller than with shyness of strangers in general, and never exceeded more than one-third of the children.

SCHOOL-CENTRED PROBLEMS

Most of the children's reactions to school were covered by the teachers' questionnaire (see Chapter 6). The parents, however, were asked about three aspects of this behaviour, namely truancy, reading difficulties, and dislike of school.

Truancy (Q.63)

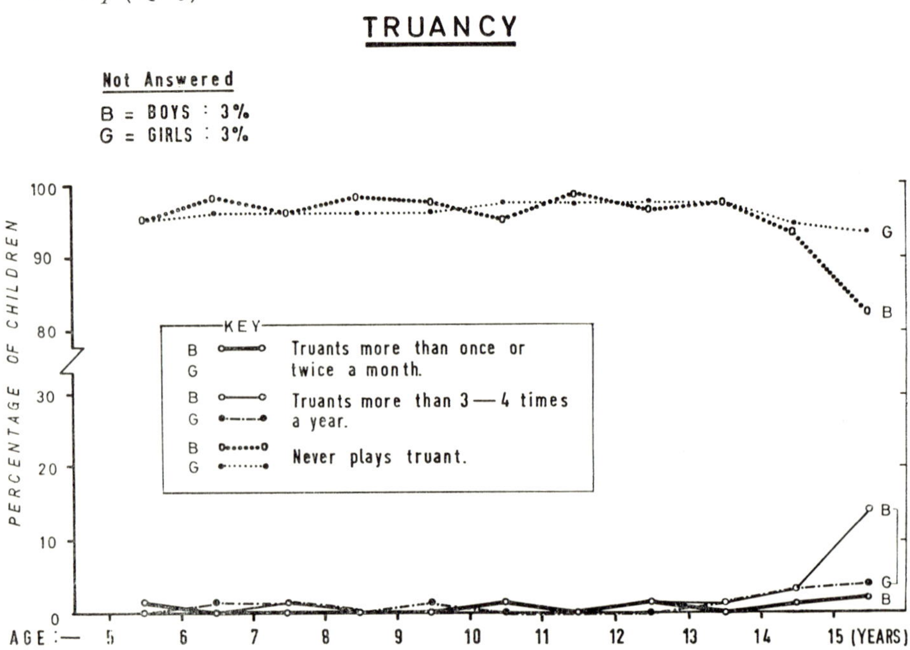

FIGURE 7

According to the parents' reports truancy was very rare: forty-one boys (13 per thousand) and thirty-one girls (10 per thousand) out of the whole sample were reported as having truanted more than three or four times a year, and only seventeen children more than once or twice a month. These estimates, however, are minimal since much successful truanting may never become known to parents if it is carried out with discretion.

Despite the small numbers it was clear that truancy was reported more frequently of children towards the end of their time at school: 49 per cent of the boy truants and 39 per cent of the girls were found among the fourteen- to fifteen-year-olds. At all ages up to fourteen there was little difference in the proportions of boys and girls, but 16 per cent of fifteen-year-old boys truanted compared with only 4 per cent of the girls. This contrasts with figures based on children attending clinics (Ackerson 1931, Mullen 1950), where boy truants predominated at all ages. The difference may well be due to selection of cases. Truants referred to child guidance clinics are usually persistent truants or children who get into trouble, e.g. for stealing, while absent from school. Such behaviour would be more characteristic of boys. Our sample deals with much milder cases. For instance, figure 7 shows that no girl played truant more than once or twice a month; only five girls were involved, and consequently the prevalence rate at each age was too small to record.

Dislike of school (Q.50)

Figure 8 overleaf makes it clear that only a minority of children—6 per cent of boys and 3 per cent of girls—were reported by their parents actively to dislike school. The proportion remained relatively constant over all ages up to twelve years, when it began to rise slowly in both sexes. It was apparent, however, that with increasing age there was a steady decrease in the proportion who showed enthusiasm for school, while the number of those with relatively neutral feelings increased.* This lessening of enthusiasm among older children was also noted by Fitt (1956) in his study of New Zealand children's attitudes to school.

At most ages, boys were more apt to show dislike of school and the overall sex difference (6 per cent of boys: 3 per cent of girls) was highly significant ($P < 0{\cdot}001$). Conversely, a higher proportion of girls (40 per cent) than boys (30 per cent) were said to like school very much, though

* It is interesting to note the similarity between the response distribution for 'attitude to school' and that shown in figure 36 for 'worrying' (see page 75).

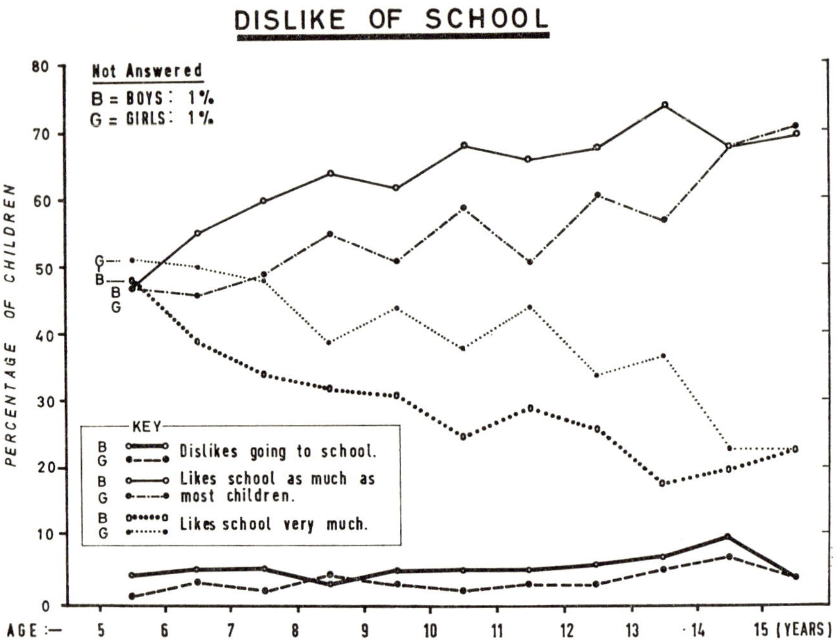

FIGURE 8

this difference was much reduced at the beginning and end of the child's school career. The sex difference in attitude to school is, once again, in close agreement with the results of other studies (Fitt 1956, Wisenthal 1965).

In this study it was unfortunately impossible to estimate the prevalence of the more extreme manifestation of 'school phobia', which usually involves actual refusal to go to school (Hersov 1961a and b, Coolidge *et al.* 1964, Frick 1964). Many of the children who disliked going to school had, nevertheless, good attendance records.* Furthermore, it has been suggested (Estes *et al.* 1956, Eisenberg 1958, Tyerman 1968) that 'school phobia' is misnamed since it is really dislike of being parted from the mother, i.e. separation anxiety, rather than a definite aversion to the school itself. Chazan (1962), however, has argued that the school situation may not be altogether unimportant in the aetiology of school phobia. In a group of thirty-three child guidance patients suffering from school phobia he found that the problem appeared during the child's first term in a new class or at

* In some of the cases interviewed in connection with the case history study it was notable that attendance was good even where the dislike of school was accompanied by psychosomatic symptoms or where force had to be employed to bring the child to school.

a new school. In our sample there was no apparent rise in the proportion disliking school among those children who were in their first year of secondary school. Since the survey took place in summer they were in their third term, however, and had had time to adjust to the change.

Reading difficulties (Q.66)

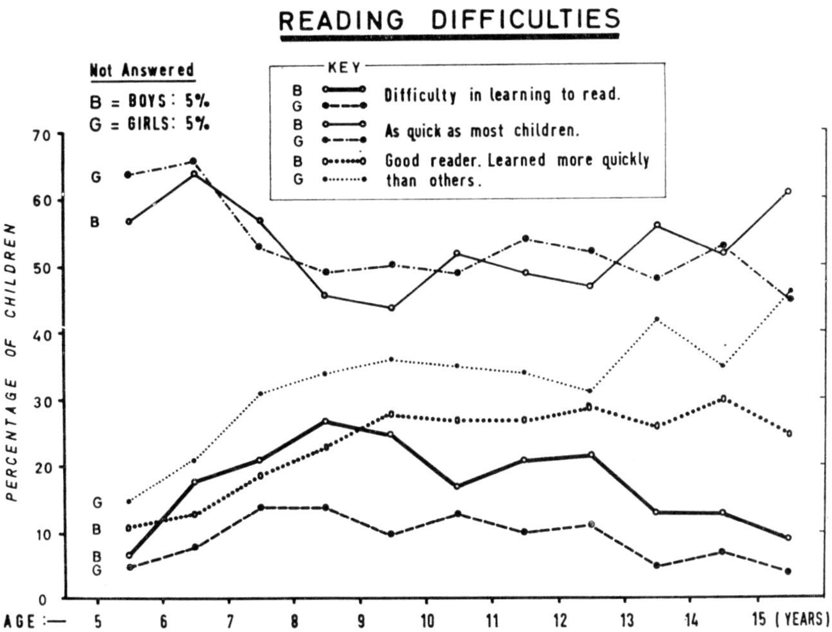

FIGURE 9

Although most children in the sample were said by their parents to have learned to read as quickly, or more quickly, than other children, there still remained a considerable number who were said to have experienced difficulty. This applied to nearly one boy in five and nearly one girl in ten. In fact, difficulty in learning to read, especially for boys, appeared to be one of the major problems reported by parents.

The age distribution of children said to have experienced this difficulty probably reflects not only the child's actual problems but also their parents' appreciation that such a problem existed. Thus, relatively few five-year-olds—5 per cent of girls and 7 per cent of boys—were said to find reading difficult. By the age of eight this group had risen to a peak of

27 per cent of boys and 14 per cent of girls. So high a proportion of eight-year-olds with reading difficulty might have led one to expect a higher prevalence rate among the younger children. However, the apparent rise probably reflects not so much a true increase in the proportion of children experiencing difficulty as the higher proportion of parents coming to realise that their children had not progressed as fast as they might wish. Most parents would be unlikely to notice any reading difficulty in a five-year-old unless the child became unhappy about it or the teacher drew their attention to it. By the age of seven or eight parents' expectations are higher and poor performance becomes less easy to overlook. It is interesting to see that the proportion of children described as good readers also rose steadily from five to nine years as the parents became increasingly aware of their childrens' abilities in this direction.

After the age of eight the proportion of children said to find difficulty in reading declined, though somewhat erratically in the case of the boys. The girls showed a more consistent decrease with increasing age.

At most ages a significantly higher proportion of boys than girls were said to find difficulty with their reading. Conversely, girls were more likely than boys at all ages to be graded as good readers who learned quickly, so that the intermediate group of those 'as quick as most children' showed little difference between the sexes.

It is noteworthy that the parents' reports discussed here which show girls as good readers more often than boys are in agreement with the results of actual testing carried out in previous studies (Pidgeon 1960, Wisenthal 1965, Pringle *et al.* 1966).

DISORDERS OF SLEEP

Restlessness in sleep (Q.71)

Figure 10 shows that the majority of children (62 per cent of boys, 63 per cent of girls) were reported as sleeping peacefully. Where restlessness was reported (25 per cent of boys, 23 per cent of girls) it was most likely to have occurred every night or else to have occurred very rarely (two or three times a year). The proportion of cases of intermediate frequencies was small: of all the children who slept restlessly, 32 per cent of the boys and 29 per cent of the girls were said to do so every night. It appears likely, therefore, that such restlessness is a long-standing characteristic of many children. The distribution varied little with age or sex.

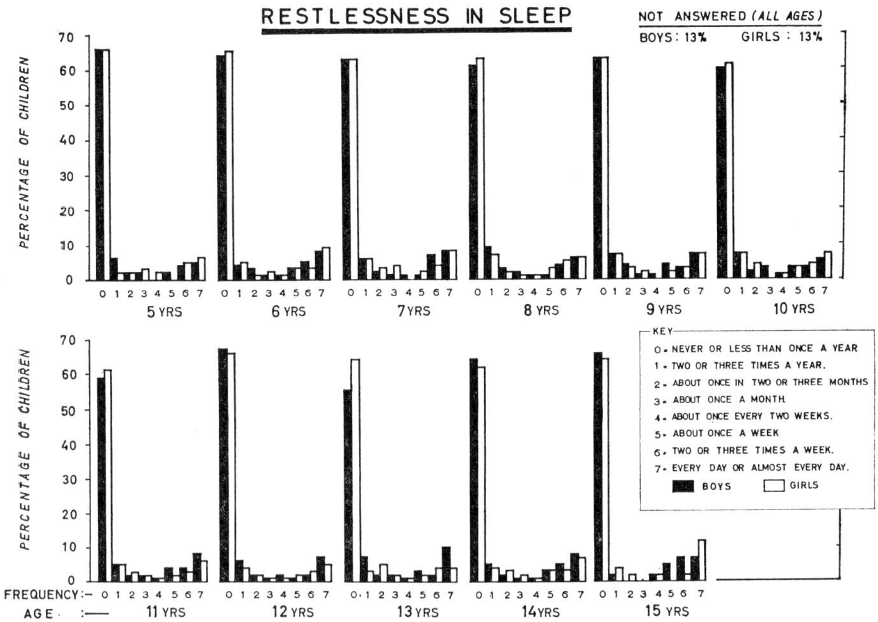

FIGURE 10

Nightmares (Q.70)

Here, again, the majority of children at all ages were described as never, or practically never, having nightmares. In the main, unpleasant dreams were said to occur only rarely: 75 per cent of the children with nightmares were recorded as having them about once in two or three months, or less often. Frequent nightmares were uncommon at all ages, being reported of only five girls and seven boys altogether. (See figure 11 overleaf.)

There was no sex difference in the reported occurrence of nightmares and, in both sexes, the proportion of children with nightmares declined with increasing age. Thus, among five-year-olds, 31 per cent of boys and 28 per cent of girls had nightmares at least two or three times a year; among ten-year-olds the corresponding proportions were 18 per cent and 22 per cent; and at the age of fourteen, there had been a further drop to 10 per cent and 14 per cent respectively. Most of this decrease appears to have occurred because of a reduction in the number of children having occasional nightmares: these may therefore either be developmental phenomena or else be reported to parents less often as the child grows older. The proportion of children reported to suffer from relatively frequent nightmares, i.e. once a fortnight or more often, showed little variation with age.

Lapouse and Monk (1958) also found a higher incidence of nightmares among six- to eight-year-olds than among older children, but Macfarlane *et al.* (1954) found that they were most common among ten-year-olds in both sexes.

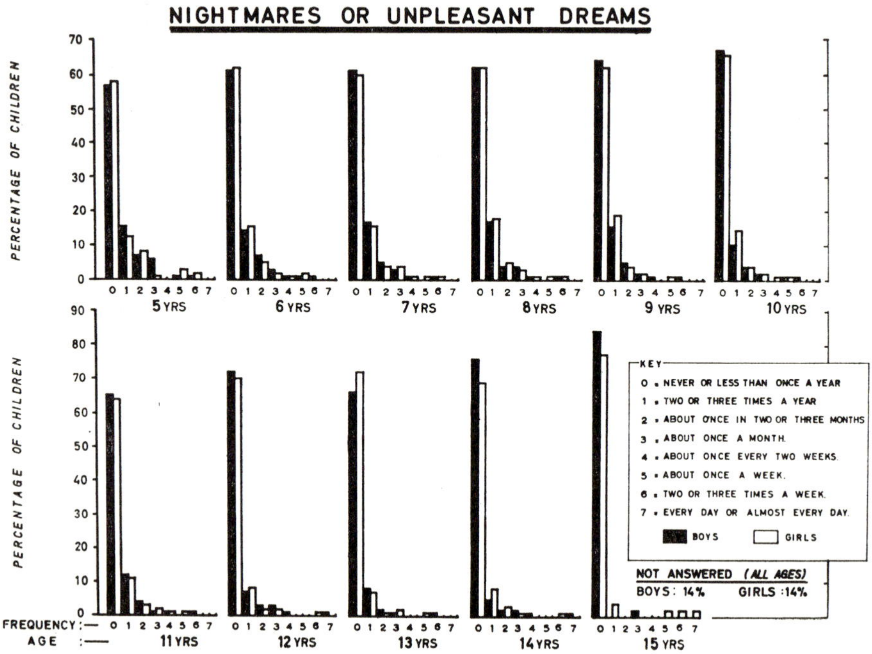

FIGURE II

Bed-wetting (Q.72)

From the age-sex data on bed-wetting (figure 12) two conclusions stand out. First, as might be expected, such episodes occurred much more frequently in the younger age group and were rare among the older children. Secondly, the reported prevalence was consistently higher among the boys than among the girls.

If we take the figures for all ages, 5 per cent of the boys and 3 per cent of the girls were said to have wet the bed at least once in two weeks; 2 per cent of the boys and 1 per cent of the girls did so nightly; at all frequencies the figure was 11 per cent of the boys and 8 per cent of the girls. Several other studies have also provided various estimates of frequency. Thus Gordon's (1942) figure was 7 per cent among 200 school-children aged five to fourteen years; Bremer's (1951) figure was 4·4 per cent of 271 children aged five to fourteen years; Gedda (1948) reported a figure of 3·6 per cent among seven-year-old children and, looking at the same age group, Hallgren (1956) found that 8 per cent of boys and 4 per cent of girls from a large, representative sample continued to wet their beds.

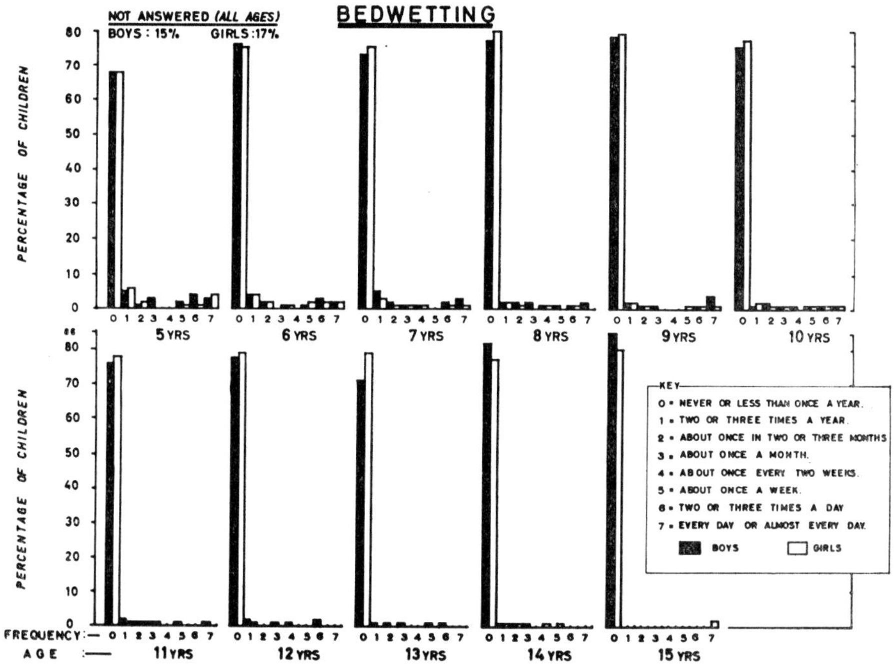

FIGURE 12

Estimates from child guidance populations are understandably higher. Addis' (1935) figure from London clinics in 1932 was 18 per cent; Kanner (1957) reported 24 per cent among his patients; Ackerson (1931) 12 per cent of girls, 14 per cent of boys. The Bakwins (1954) found that 26 per cent of a thousand children attending a general out-patient clinic at Bellvue Hospital in New York were enuretic.

The influence of age on reported frequency emerges clearly from several studies. Michaels and Goodman (1934) reported that about 9·2 per cent of eight-year-old normal children and 3·9 per cent of ten-year-olds at an American Recreation Camp were still bed-wetters. McConachie (Ministry of Education 1954–5), a school medical officer, found in a sample of 1600 school children that the proportion wetting their beds more than once a week fell from 10 per cent at five years to 2·5 per cent at thirteen or over. In York, Bransby *et al.* (1955) reported that whereas 18 per cent of five-year-olds were bed-wetters, this proportion fell to 9 per cent at the age of nine to ten years and to 2·5 per cent of the children over the age of twelve. In their Newcastle survey, Miller *et al.* (1960) found that 9 per cent of their sample were still wetting their beds 'either habitually or often enough for parents to take regular precautions' when they were five; by the time they were nine the proportion had fallen to 7 per cent. A National Survey (Blomfield and Douglas 1956) identified 4 per cent of six-year-old boys and girls as regular bed-wetters; for girls, this figure had fallen to 2 per cent by the age of seven and three-quarters, though the proportion of boys remained constant. Occasional bed-wetting fell from 8 per cent of boys and 5 per cent of girls at six years to 5 per cent and 4 per cent respectively at the age of seven and three-quarters.

This decline of frequency with age is not so apparent among the child guidance population (Barbour *et al.* 1963). Kanner (1957), for example, has reported a peak prevalence between the ages of eight to eleven years but he also provides the likely explanation for this discrepancy: 'It means that its persistence until then has made parents and referring physicians aware of the need for psychiatric consideration of the problem'.

The clear sex difference emerging from our data has been confirmed by several other investigators. Bransby (1955) found that four- to ten-year-old girls exhibited a frequency which was only 85 per cent of that of the boys. Blomfield and Douglas (1956) reported that the rate for girls was only 60 per cent that of the boys. McConachie (Ministry of Education 1954–5) estimated that, by the age of ten, the number of enuretic boys was double that of the girls, and Hallgren (1956) also detected a significantly higher rate among boys. Of the children attending child guidance clinics, Kanner (1957) reported 62 per cent of bed-wetters to be boys.

ANTI-SOCIAL BEHAVIOUR

Since our questionnaire was designed to be administered to the parents of presumably normal children, it did not attempt to provide a comprehensive coverage of extremely anti-social or delinquent behaviour. Such behaviour might be expected to be rare in such a population; parents would be unlikely to provide information about it and, indeed, might well have been antagonized if the questions had referred to it. Only a limited number of items were therefore included; these were destructiveness, stealing, lying, playing truant and wandering from home.

Destructiveness (Q.45)

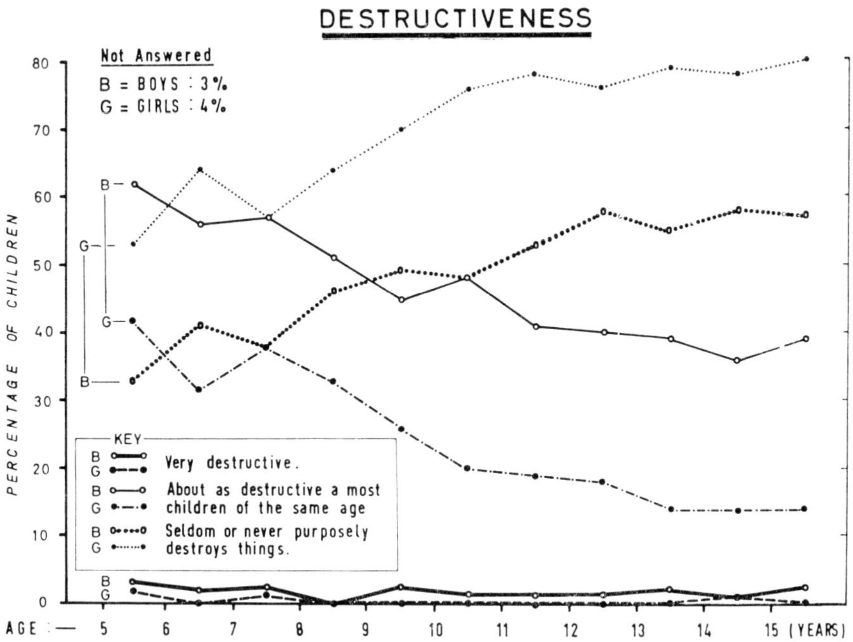

FIGURE 13

Figure 13 shows that a very small minority of children were considered 'very destructive' at any age; in all, this applied to only thirteen girls (4 per thousand) and forty-three boys (13 per thousand). The reported behaviour pattern of the remainder was of the 'developmental' type, with mild destructiveness at its peak among the five-year-olds, where it was reported by the parents of 62 per cent of the boys and 42 per cent of the girls, then falling to a minimum of 14 per cent of girls and 36 per cent of boys at the age of fourteen. Conversely, an increasing proportion of children were reported free from destructiveness with seniority, reaching a peak of 30 per cent among the fifteen-year-old girls. The same trend has been reported by Macfarlane *et al.* (1954) for normal children, and by Ackerson (1931) and by Grant (1958) for child guidance patients. Boys were more likely than girls to be rated as 'very destructive' at most ages and a similar and even more consistent sex difference was clearly apparent for 'mild' destructiveness.

Stealing (Q.51)

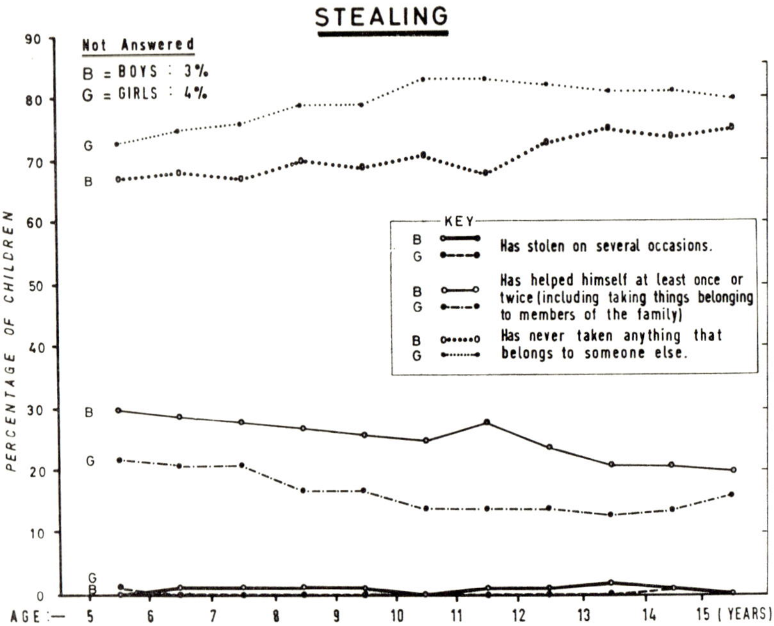

FIGURE 14

The question about stealing was of necessity worded with some care and referred to past as well as present events. From the answers, it is clear that the parents of the great majority of children denied that any degree of stealing ever took place. Only very few children, nearly all boys, were reported to have stolen on several occasions. Other workers who have discussed stealing as a problem encountered in clinic or court naturally report higher figures (Kanner 1957, Ackerson 1931, Bakwin and Bakwin 1954). In the milder category of 'helping himself' boys again predominated, with a reported prevalence rate of 29 per cent compared with 17 per cent for girls. In both sexes stealing was recorded at its peak among five- to six-year-olds and then declined with increasing age.

Lying (Q.49)

Figure 15 shows that most of the children were believed by their mothers to tell 'an occasional fib', but relatively few were reported to 'tell deliberate

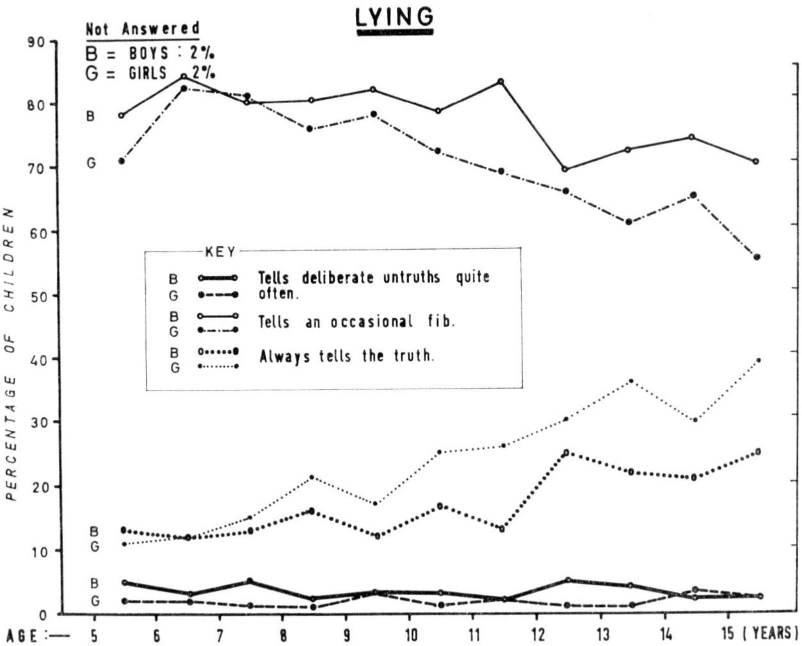

FIGURE 15

untruths quite often: The distinction between 'fibs' and 'deliberate untruth' is, of course, subjective, depending very much on the mother's own frame of reference as well as on the child's behaviour. 'An occasional fib', however, probably signifies less parental concern over the behaviour.

Truthfulness became more frequently reported with increasing age; 39 per cent of girls and 25 per cent of boys of fifteen were believed always to tell the truth compared with 12 per cent of both sexes at the age of six. The apparent increase in veracity with age came at the expense of the occasional fibbers rather than that of the frequent liars. There was no relation between age and the reported telling of deliberate untruths, which maintained an average of 3 per cent for boys and 2 per cent for girls. At all ages, girls were less likely than boys to be described as telling either deliberate untruths or occasional fibs.

In their sample of normal children Macfarlane *et al.* (1954) found a decrease in reported lying after the age of five or six. The picture from the child guidance clinic, however, is quite different. Grant (1958) reported an increase of lying among older children attending the Maudsley Hospital; according to Ackerson (1931) lying, usually of a protective nature, increased with age in both sexes up to the age of eight or nine, after which age it tended to decrease among boys but to increase among girls until the age of seventeen.

Disobedience (Q.62)

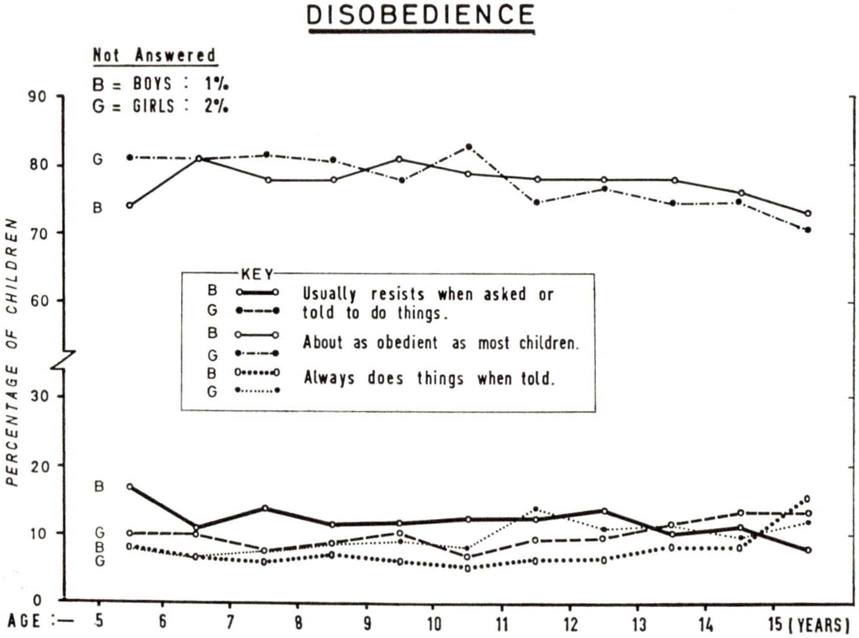

FIGURE 16

Perhaps surprisingly, the pattern of reported obedient behaviour differed markedly from that of truthfulness. The paragons who always did as they were told comprised only 10 per cent of the girls and 8 per cent of the boys, not too low a figure if we accept Kanner's view of 'complete obedience' as the expression of pathological submissiveness resulting from suppression of spontaneity and initiative.

A further 10 per cent of the girls and 13 per cent of the boys were reported as 'usually resisting when asked or told to do things'; and approximately 80 per cent of the children were considered by their parents 'about as obedient as most children'. The age and sex trends within this pattern were unremarkable.

The most relevant information in the psychiatric literature concerns the more severe manifestation of 'negativism' rather than disobedience. Reynolds (1928) and Levy and Tulchin (1932) found the peak age for negativism to be between the second and third years, but Macfarlane *et al.*

(1954) estimated that children of three to six were most prone to this behaviour. On the other hand, Griffiths (1952) and Ackerson (1931) put the peak period at nine to eleven years. No marked sex difference appeared in these studies, though on the whole boys were considered to be more refractory.

Wandering (Q.60)

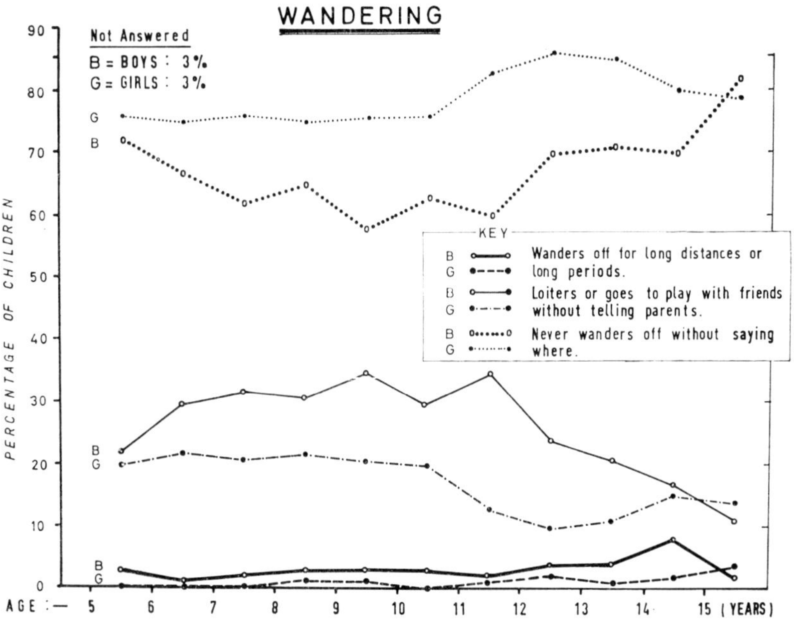

FIGURE 17

It is evident from figure 17 that the majority of children in this sample were not given to wandering. Where wandering was reported, it was more likely to have occurred among boys (4 per cent) than among girls (1 per cent). This was also true of the more moderate category, comprising children who were apt to loiter or go off to play with friends without telling their parents. A change in reported behaviour occurred at adolescence in both sexes. On the one hand, there was an increase in the small number of children who 'wander off for long distances or long periods'. On the other hand, the number of children who were said never to wander also increased, while the number in the middle category fell. This change might, of course, merely reflect diminished anxiety on the part of parents about their children's whereabouts as the children grew older.

In their study of normal children, Macfarlane *et al.* (1954) found that reports of 'truancy from home' ceased at the age of seven years: 'It was no longer regarded as truancy by mothers when the children were old enough, in the mother's eyes, to protect themselves and enjoy more freedom'. Among children attending psychiatric clinics in New York Ackerson (1931) reported 'truancy from home' in 20 per cent of white boys and 13 per cent of white girls, with a maximum age frequency for boys at ten to twelve years and for girls at seventeen or eighteen.*

PHYSICAL DISORDERS

Physical health was, on the whole, confined to a separate part of the questionnaire, which is described in Chapter 5. There were some types of physical problem, however, which could reflect psychological as well as somatic disturbance. These were included in the eight-point scale in the behavioural section of the questionnaire and consisted of 'constipation', 'headaches', 'stomach pains', 'vomiting', 'diarrhoea' and 'soiling'. No attempt has been made to differentiate the items into psychogenic and somatogenic categories. This clearly would have been impossible for the information available; it is often difficult enough for the clinician.

In general, these items show a similar type of distribution, with the proportion of cases reported falling as the frequency of the behaviour increases. Most of the children with physical complaints exhibited them only at rare intervals. There was, however, some distinction in that headaches, constipation and stomach pains occurred very much more commonly at all frequencies than did diarrhoea and vomiting, while soiling was very uncommon. A further noteworthy point lies in the reported increase in the prevalence of monthly stomach pains, headaches and, to some extent, vomiting, among adolescent girls.

Constipation (Q.68)

From the histograms shown in figure 18 it can be seen that more than half the sample (56 per cent of girls; 62 per cent of boys) were said never to

* These very high figures very probably reflect the way in which Ackerson's patients were recruited. Children who wander are more likely to be open to encouragement to delinquent behaviour and may also come from less stable environments. On both counts they would be more liable to official intervention in their affairs and consequently to referral to a 'behaviour clinic'.

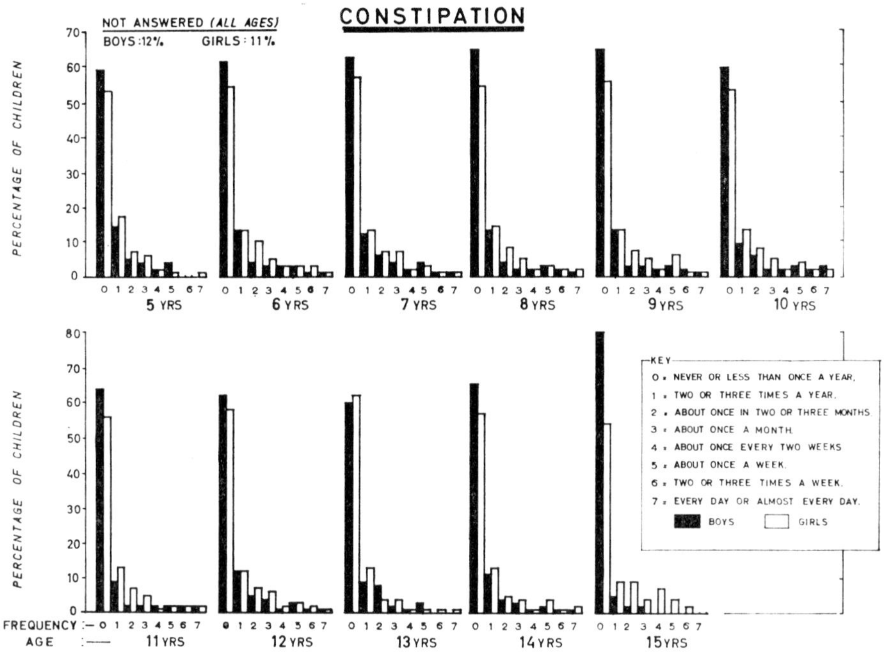

FIGURE 18

suffer from constipation. Among those who did, prevalence fell steadily as frequency increased: 40 per cent of the girls and 44 per cent of the boys reported as constipated suffered such episodes only two or three times a year, and it appeared to be a chronic condition in only a small proportion of cases. Over the whole range of frequency, girls were more likely than boys ($P < 0{\cdot}001$) to be reported as suffering from constipation. Most of this difference, however, occurred in the groups with occasional rather than frequent constipation. There was also a tendency for reports of constipation to decrease among older children, though there is no way of assessing whether the change concerns the child's habits or the mother's knowledge of them.

Diarrhoea (Q.75)

Figure 19 (page 58) depicts a physical complaint which was very infrequently reported. Only 17 per cent of boys and 14 per cent of girls were said to suffer from diarrhoea, and not more than 18 per cent of those experienced attacks of diarrhoea more than two or three times a year. In

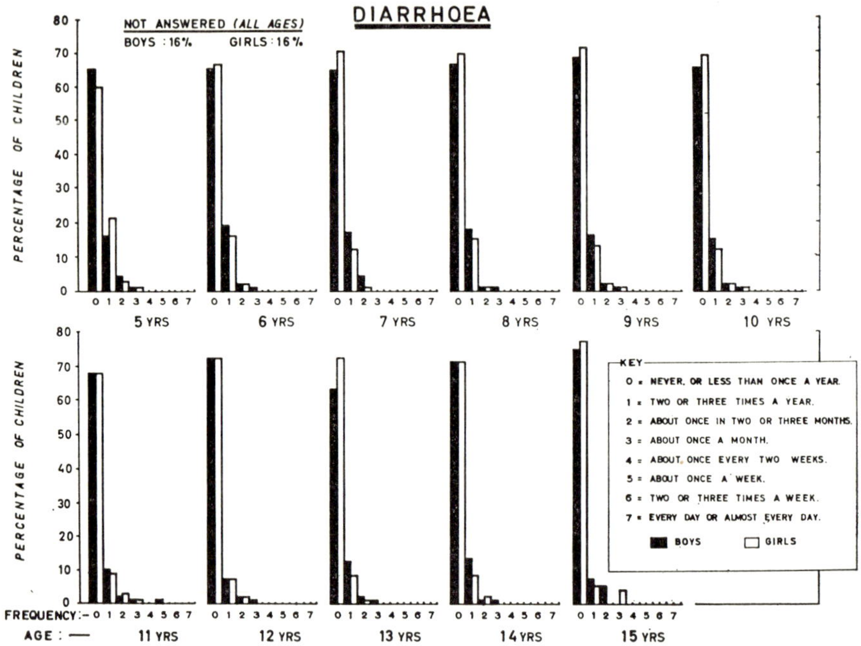

FIGURE 19

each sex there was a tendency for prevalence to fall with increasing age, albeit rather slowly and irregularly. At all ages except five years, girls were slightly more likely to suffer from diarrhoea than were boys.

Soiling (Q.76)

As might be expected of a school-age sample of children, only a very small proportion were reported to be soiling themselves at all. This may, of course, be an under-estimate of the true prevalence, as the parents of 18 per cent of the children did not complete the item. Figure 20 shows that soiling was significantly more likely to occur among boys (4 per cent) than girls (2 per cent) ($P < 0{\cdot}001$). Among the children who did soil themselves, boys were also likely to do so more frequently than girls: 62 per cent of the boys who soiled were recorded as doing so more than two or three times a year, whereas the corresponding figure for girls was only 44 per cent. Among the fifty-three children who were reported to soil themselves once a week or more often, forty (75 per cent) were boys, and the same sex ratio (1:3) was found among the children who were said to soil every day.

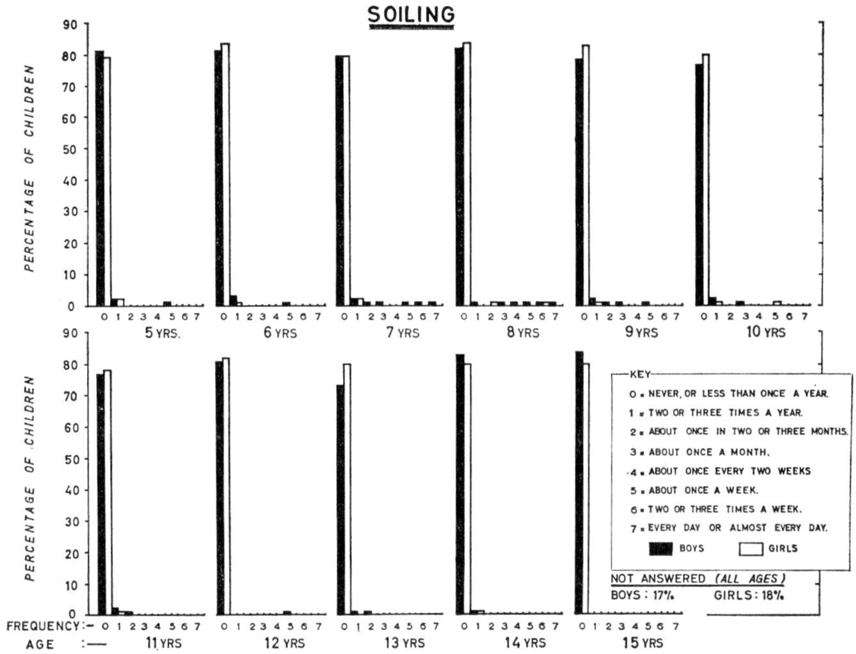

FIGURE 20

Reports of soiling were extremely rare among children over the age of ten. Among the younger girls soiling was said to occur most often at five, though, even then, it was extremely rare and was likely to take the form of infrequent 'accidents'. Among the boys the recorded peak both for prevalence and for frequency was from seven to nine years of age.

Pains in stomach (Q.73)

The pattern illustrated in figure 21 (page 60) is not dissimilar from that shown by the distribution of reported headaches (see page 62): the recorded prevalence tends to decrease as the frequency of occurrence rises, and girls who have started their periods present a distinctive picture. From the age of twelve years onwards, an increasing proportion of girls were said to complain of pains every month, which became the most commonly reported frequency. Up to the age of ten, only 4 per cent of girls suffered from pains in the stomach; among the twelve- to thirteen-year-olds this figure had risen to 15 per cent; and by fourteen and fifteen years of age the proportion had risen to nearly one in every four girls. This is in agreement with the findings of other epidemiological studies of adolescent girls: Heald *et al.* (1957) reported that 37 per cent of girls of sixteen to seventeen and a half in a New England school suffered from abdominal cramps; Van Laar *et al.* (1962) found about one in six of a sample of older adolescent Dutch schoolgirls lost at least one day's schooling because of menstrual troubles, including pain. Since the reported rate for boys remained constant at 3 per cent, it appears likely that the category of 'pains in the stomach' is being swollen by the inclusion of some girls' period pains. Information on menstruation was obtained independently from the health

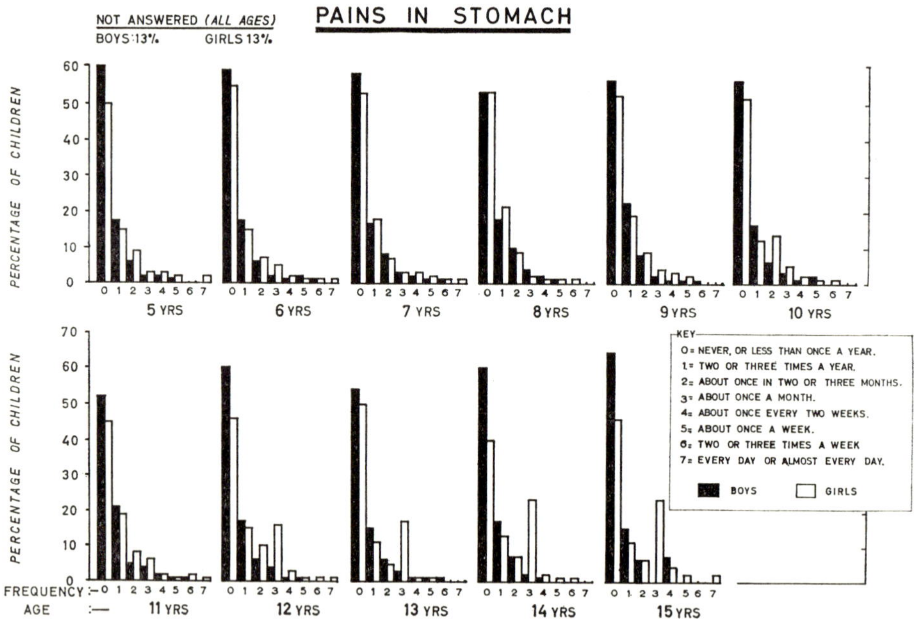

FIGURE 21

section of the questionnaire, and a comparison showed that seventy (36 per cent) of the 195 girls aged eleven to fifteen who were reported to suffer from monthly stomach pains in answer to Question 73 were also said to complain of pain during their periods. Even if these cases are excluded, however, a relatively high proportion of 11 per cent of girls over ten years old were still reported to suffer pain once a month.

The prevalence of pains reported as occurring more often than once a month is still slightly higher among the girls (5 per cent) than among the boys (3 per cent), but there is very little variation with age.

Vomiting (Q.74)

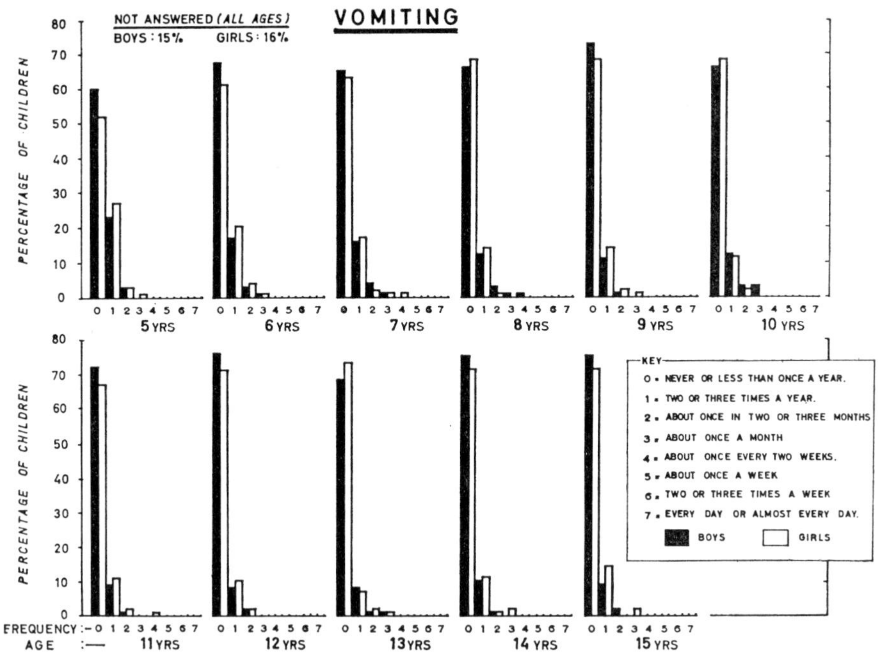

FIGURE 22

Reports of vomiting were relatively rare, with only 16 per cent of boys and 17 per cent of girls recorded as vomiting even once during a year. As figure 22 shows, most children did not vomit more than two or three times a year. Only nine girls and eight boys were recorded as vomiting more than once a month, and all but four of these only did so less than once a week.

Very infrequent vomiting, i.e. two or three times a year, was most common among the youngest children in the sample and declined with age. More frequent vomiting was too rare to allow for age comparisons. A pattern of monthly vomiting developed in girls after the age of twelve years. Otherwise there did not appear to be any specific sex variation in the distributions.

Headaches (Q.69)

More than half of the total children in the sample (54 per cent of boys; 57 per cent of girls) were reported to suffer from headaches at least two or three times a year. Such an overall figure is, however, a little misleading as the proportion of children who had headaches rose steadily with older children. Thus, although only about one-third of the five-year-olds were said to have headaches, this symptom was reported of two-thirds of children aged fourteen or fifteen. In the majority of cases the headaches appeared to be infrequent, occurring only once in two or three months or less often. In general, the proportion of these children declined as the frequency of occurrence increased. There was, however, one exception. Among the girls aged twelve or more, at least as many monthly headaches were reported as were those occurring more infrequently, once in two or three months. This was not so among the boys and probably reflects a tendency for headaches to be associated with menstruation or an expectation that they will occur at such a time. Very few children were said to suffer from headaches more than once a week, and most of those who did were over ten years old.

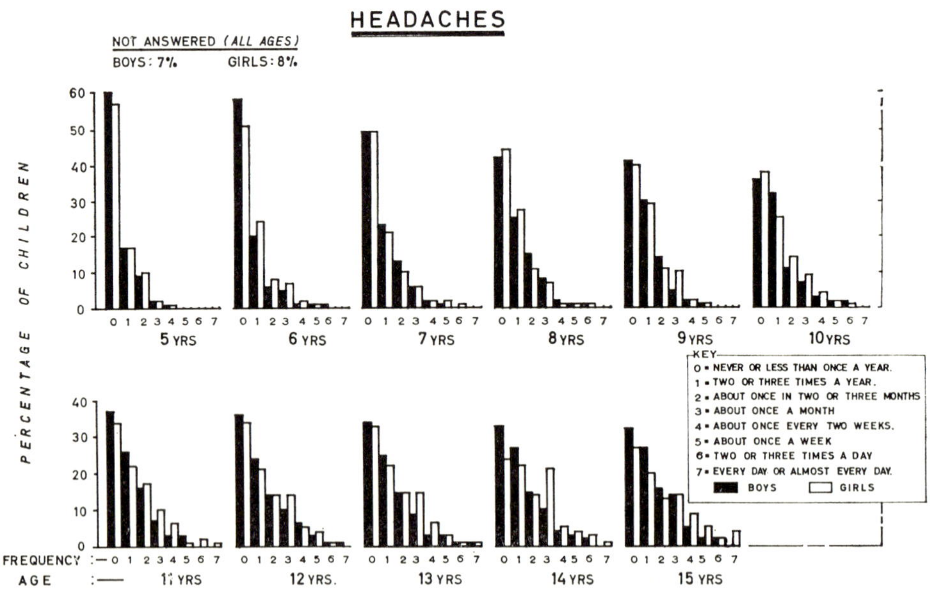

FIGURE 23

In general, the older children were more likely to be reported as having frequent headaches. Thus, among the girls 12 per cent of those aged between eleven and fifteen were said to have headaches at least once a fortnight, compared with only 5 per cent of the five- to ten-year-olds ($P < 0{\cdot}001$). A similar picture appeared among the boys, where the figures were 9 per cent and 4 per cent respectively ($P < 0{\cdot}001$). In pre-adolescence there was no apparent sex difference in prevalence, but among the older children girls were likely to have headaches reported more often than boys.

PSYCHOMOTOR BEHAVIOUR

Restlessness and under-activity (Q.58)

Both extreme responses on this item were regarded as indicating possible problems of behaviour. These responses are, of course, coloured by the reporting parent's experience and expectations. As Macfarlane *et al.* (1954) have pointed out, it is difficult, even in an interview, to separate reports of over-activity from 'the mother's state of health, the home living-space, and legitimate activities provided for the child'.

a. *Restlessness* Reports of restlessness and fidgety behaviour were by no means uncommon: in all, 20 per cent of boys and 14 per cent of girls were described in this way. Boys were more likely than girls to be

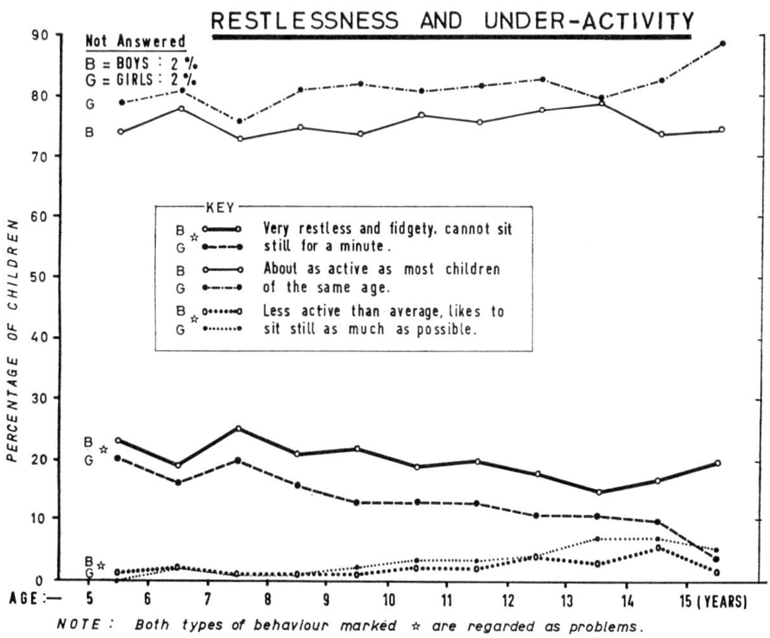

FIGURE 24

reported as restless and, as can be seen in figure 24 (page 63), this difference existed in each age group. Indeed, up to the age of thirteen the age distribution curves for each sex followed a very similar pattern. In both sexes reports of restlessness reached their peak among seven-year-olds (25 per cent of boys 20 per cent of girls) and then dropped steadily except for the rise found among the oldest boys. Macfarlane *et al.* (1954), dealing with normal children, and Ackerson (1931) with a clinic population reported a decline in restlessness with age. Ackerson also found the peak prevalence rate among seven-year-olds. Macfarlane suggests that the highest rate occurred in the pre-school period, but did find a subsidiary peak among seven-year-old boys.

b. Under-activity Only a relatively small proportion of the children (3 per cent of girls, 2 per cent of boys) were described as 'less active than average'. Figure 24 shows that this proportion tended to increase with age, reaching its peak in both sexes at the age of fourteen (7 per cent of girls, 6 per cent of boys). There was no indication of any sex difference in reported prevalence.

Tics (Q.64)

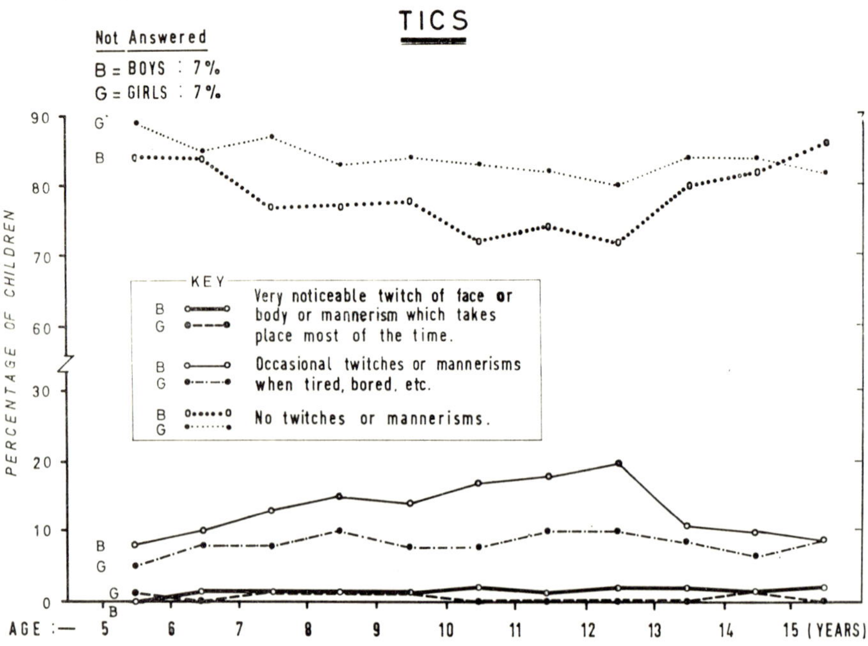

FIGURE 25

Even in terms of the fairly wide definitions used tics were rarely reported, especially among girls; only fifteen girls and forty boys were said to have noticeable and persistent twitches. This low prevalence is not unexpected, as Pasamanick and Kawi (1956) could only find eighty-three children with tics recorded as having attended a busy child psychiatric clinic over a period of thirty years. The large majority of children (80 per cent) were recorded as manifesting no twitches or mannerisms,* but in a fairly substantial minority some twitches and mannerisms became evident when the child was tired or bored.

The prevalence of tics among boys remained relatively constant at between 1 to 2 per cent for all ages from six to fifteen. Among the girls there was little variation up to the age of nine, but among ten- to thirteen-year-olds only two cases of tics were reported out of a total of 1165 children.

Boys were more likely than girls both to suffer from tics and to be reported as showing occasional twitches or mannerisms. In the moderate category the size of the group increased with age to reach a peak of 20 per cent among twelve-year-old boys before falling again. The proportion of girls, however, remained relatively constant at from 8 to 10 per cent for all ages from six to fifteen.

Nail-biting (Q.80)

It is important to think of intensity as well as frequency in assessing the distribution of nail-biting. At all ages it is illustrated by a U-shaped distribution: either the children did not bite their nails at all or else they did so very frequently. At nearly all ages girls were slightly more likely to bite their nails than were boys. In all, 25 per cent of boys and 29 per cent of girls were said to bite their nails at least two or three times a year; of these 53 per cent of the boys and 48 per cent of the girls did so every day. Previous assessments have varied according to the age of the children studied and the definition of nail-biting adopted but, as table 5 on page 66 shows, they have all shown that it is by no means a rare phenomenon.

Prevalence showed some variation with age. Daily nail-biting was least common among five-year-olds (9 per cent of girls and 6 per cent of boys). The highest rates of daily nail-biting occurred among boys at nine years (18 per cent) and girls at eleven (19 per cent). (See figure 26, page 66.)

* For convenience, the vertical scale in figure 25 has been broken and this must be noted in comparing the three curves for each sex.

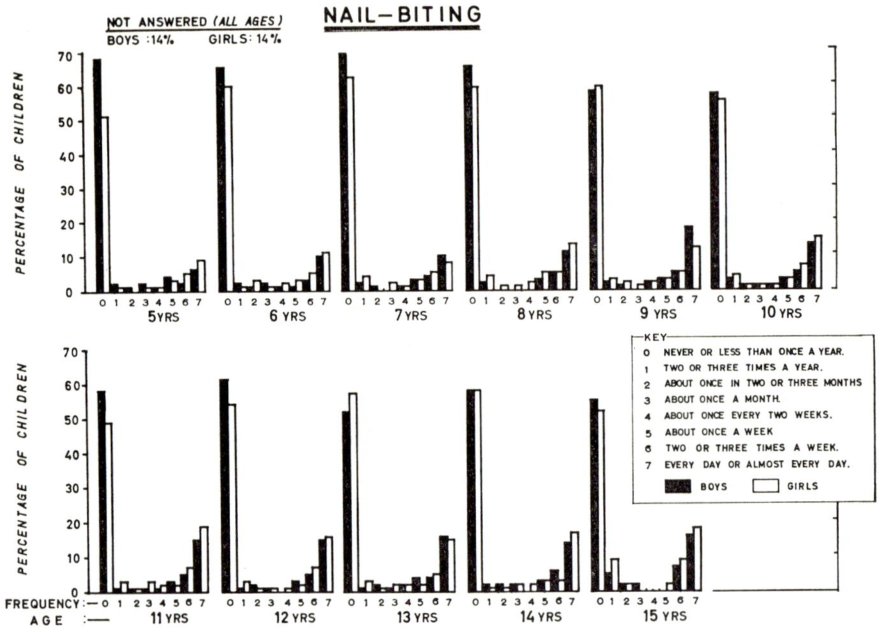

FIGURE 26

TABLE 5. *Results of some previous surveys on incidence of nail-biting among children*

Investigator	*Number of children*	*Age-range* (years)	*Location*	Incidence found		
				Boys %	*Girls* %	*Sexes not separated* %
Billig (1941)	223	8–16	School	32	41	–
Birch (1955)	4000	5–18	School	–	–	51
Lapouse and Monk (1964)	482	6–12	Mother's report	–	–	27
Malone and Massler (1952)	4587	5–18	School	–	–	41
Valentine (1956)	272	5–15	School	–	–	45
Wechsler (1931)	3000	1–17	School and pre-school	34*	33*	–
Macfarlane *et al* (1954)	Varied from 116 at 1¾ yrs. to 41 at 14 yrs.†	1–14	Special survey group	17	23	–
Ackerson (1931)	5000	2–18	Psychiatric clinic	11	16	–

* *Wechsler covered an age-range from one to seventeen years, but these figures have been calculated from his more detailed information on the school age (five to sixteen years) children only.*

† *This was a longitudinal study of one group of children re-examined yearly, but the sample was reduced considerably over time.*

Thumb-sucking (Q.81)

Like nail-biting, thumb-sucking was reported as occurring either very frequently or not at all: 85 per cent of the children aged five to ten who sucked their thumbs did so two or three times a week or more often, and the corresponding proportion between the ages of eleven and fifteen was 76 per cent. The recorded prevalence of thumb-sucking in each sex fell with age, though at all ages girls were more likely than boys to suck their

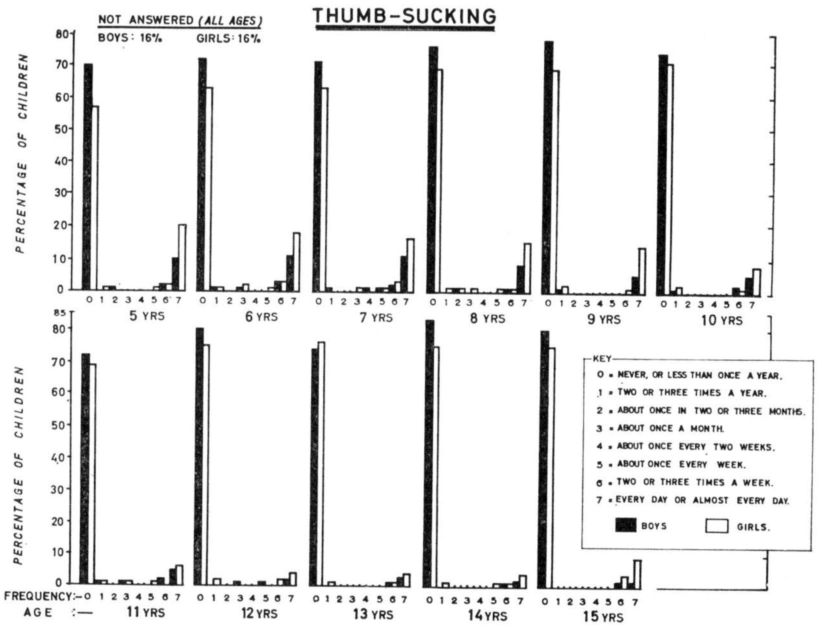

FIGURE 27

thumbs every day. Thus, while 20 per cent of girls and 10 per cent of boys were daily thumb-suckers at five years old, these proportions had fallen to 8 per cent of girls and 5 per cent of boys aged ten and were halved again by the time the children were fourteen.

It has been shown (Gesell and Ilg 1946, Macfarlane *et al.* 1954, Traisman and Traisman 1958) that the peak age for thumb-sucking is in the pre-school phase of development; the present sample, therefore, covers only the tail of the distribution.

EMOTIONAL BEHAVIOUR

Crying (Q.77)

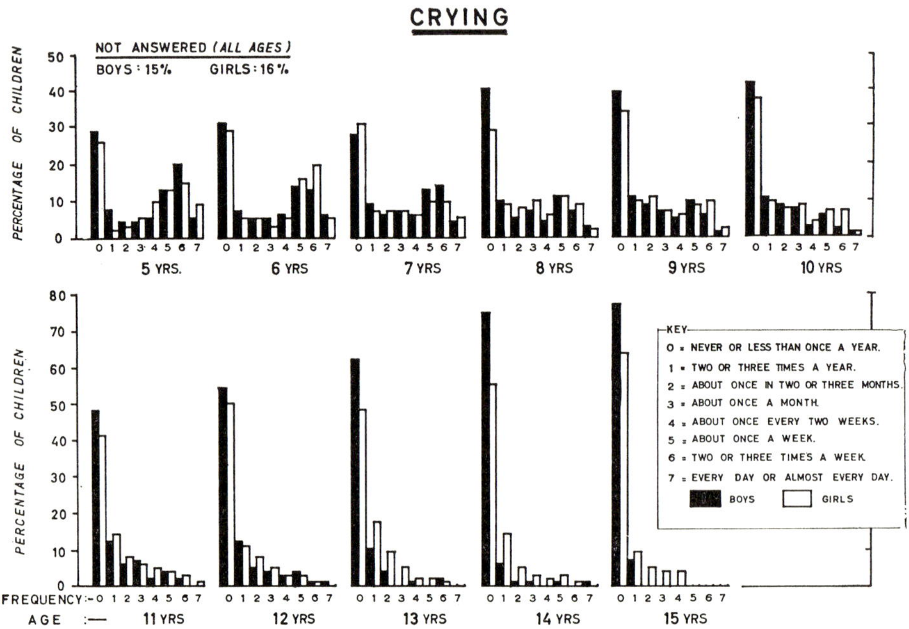

FIGURE 28

Crying, as might be expected, was closely associated with age. As the children became older there was not only a steady increase in the proportion who were reported as never crying but also a marked change in the frequency of any crying which was noted. Among the five-year-olds, the distribution is almost U-shaped. Approximately one third of the children were reported as not crying at all and 25 per cent as crying at least two or three times a week. Gradually the pattern changed as the children grew older so that, by the age of eleven crying was most likely to occur with relative infrequency. The proportion of children who never cried also rose from 41 per cent of girls and 48 per cent of boys aged eleven to 64 per cent of girls and 77 per cent of boys at the age of fifteen.

Contrary to popular belief, there was little tendency among the younger children for girls to cry more than boys. Among the older children, however, the gap between the sexes widened steadily.

Whining (Q.57)

In both sexes, complaining and whining 'a lot' was relatively uncommon and, on the whole, was reported less frequently as the children grew older. Among the five-year-olds 7 per cent of both boys and girls were said to complain a lot but by the age of thirteen this figure had fallen to 3 per cent.

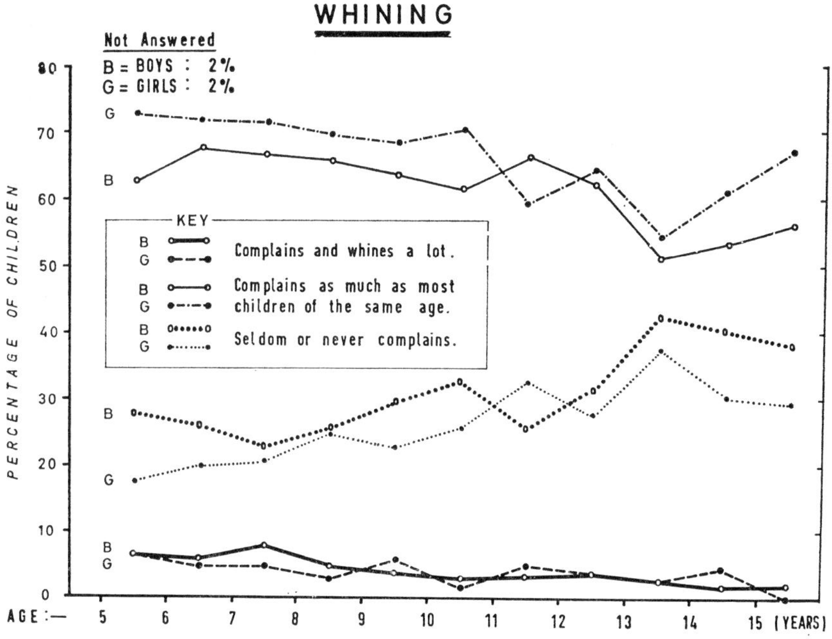

FIGURE 29

At the same time, the number of paragons who 'seldom or never complained' was increasing.

Boys, on the whole, appeared to complain less than girls; this was due to the greater proportion of girls recorded as being in the middle category. Reports of frequent complaints and whining were made equally about both boys and girls.

Sulking (Q.78)

The distribution pattern for sulking can be seen to differ from that of whining and complaining since the majority of children were recorded as never sulking. Frequent sulking was uncommon and disappeared almost entirely among the boys after the age of eight. The numbers of children said to sulk infrequently were also small and the proportion said to sulk two or three times a year rose slightly as the children grew older, up to the age of thirteen.

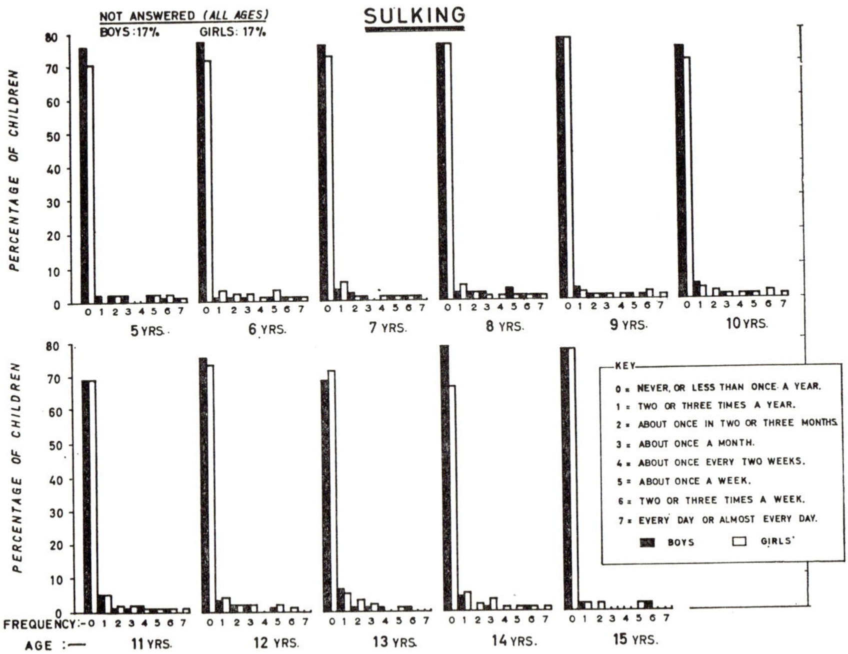

FIGURE 30

Irritability (Q.52)

About three-quarters of the children were considered to be cross occasionally and 11 per cent of both boys and girls were said to be 'very irritable'. Irritability was not associated with sex, and marked irritability showed no consistent change with age. Reports of placidity increased as the children became older, with an accompanying reduction in the number of children reported as occasionally becoming cross. Macfarlane *et al.* (1954) and Ackerson (1931) reported similar findings.

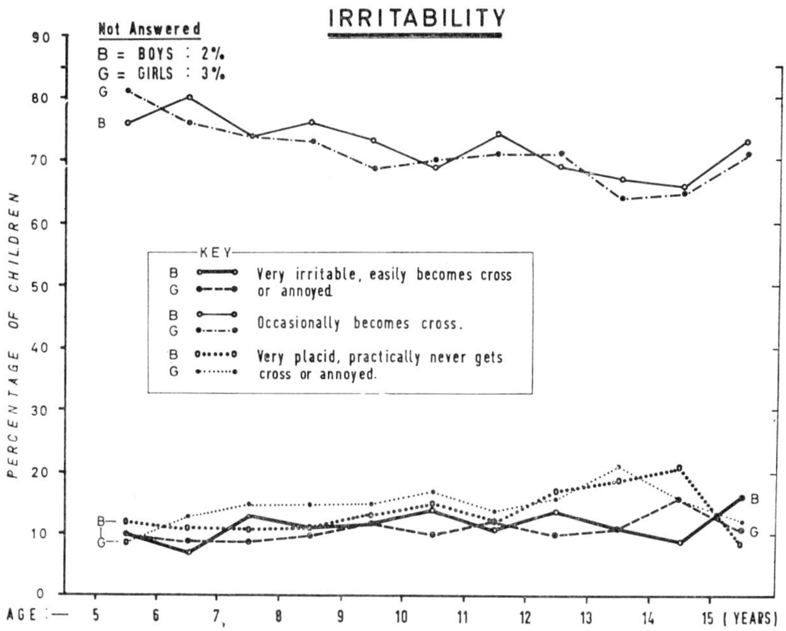

FIGURE 31

Temper tantrums (Q.79)

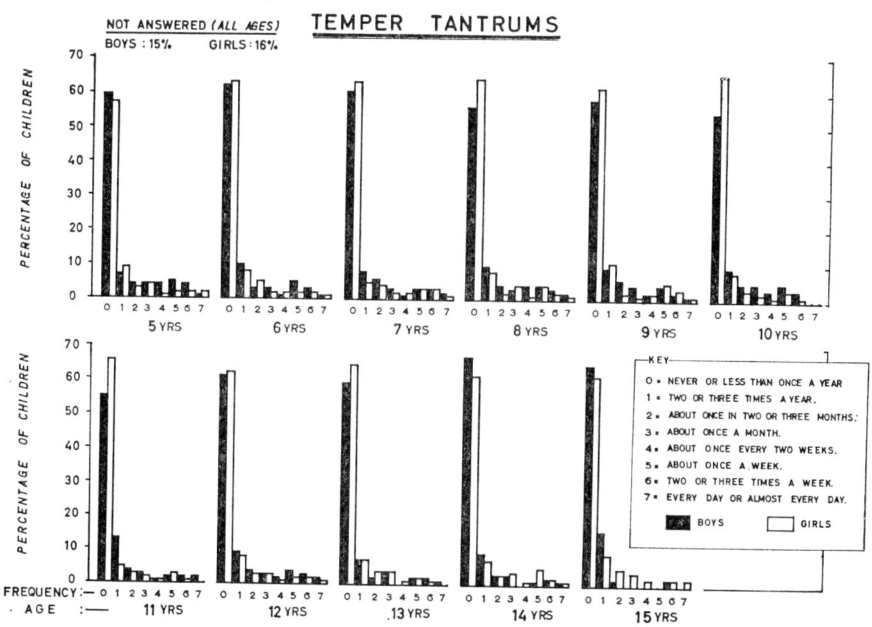

FIGURE 32

Figure 32 (page 71) shows frequent tantrums were relatively uncommon. Nevertheless, 6 per cent of the girls and 7 per cent of the boys were reported as having tantrums at least once a week, and 26 per cent of the boys and 20 per cent of the girls as having tantrums at least two or three times a year. The prevalence of frequent tantrums was associated with age in each sex. Among the boys, 10 per cent of five-year-olds were said to be having tantrums weekly or more often: this figure fell steadily with age to 2 per cent by the age of fifteen. Among the girls, the corresponding figure did not drop until after the age of nine and there was another up-swing among the fourteen- and fifteen-year-olds. Other writers (Bakwin and Bakwin 1954, Kanner 1957, Macfarlane *et al.* 1954) have suggested that the peak prevalence of tantrums occurs in pre-school days, probably just before the third birthday.

In our sample, more boys than girls were reported as having tantrums except in the fourteen- to fifteen-year age group.

Bitter quarrels with other children (Q.82)

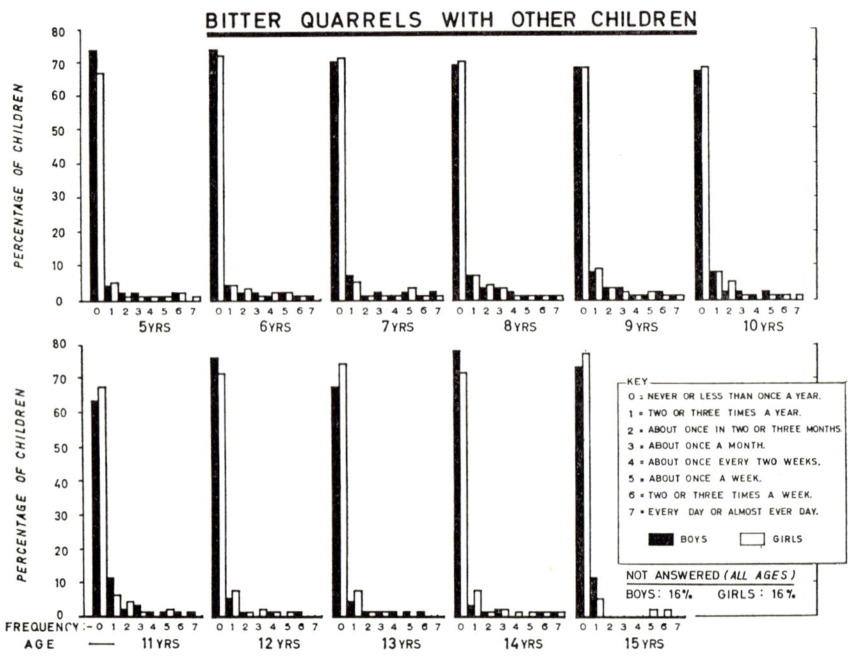

FIGURE 33

At all ages it was uncommon to find quarrelling with other children recorded: 70 per cent of the sample, or 84 per cent of those whose parents answered this question, were reported either never to quarrel with other children or only to do so less than once a year. Among those who quarrelled more often, nearly half were recorded as doing so only two or three times a year. As figure 33 shows, reports of frequent quarrelling with other children were rare, particularly after the age of eleven. There was no significant difference between the sexes.

Jealousy (Q.59)

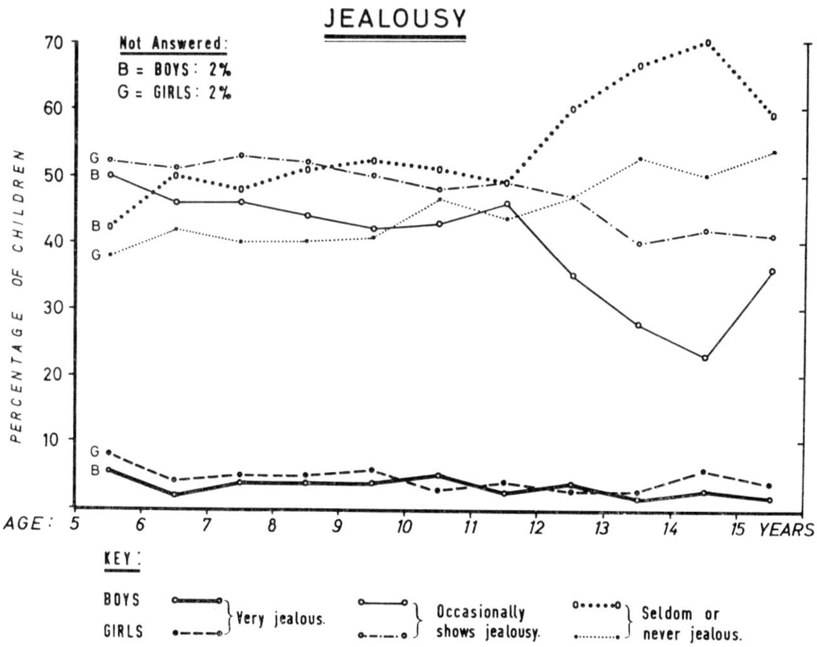

FIGURE 34

Only 4 per cent of the boys in the sample and 5 per cent of the girls were described as 'very jealous'. In both sexes jealousy was most prevalent among the five-year-olds. This applied both to acute jealousy and to mild occasional jealousy. After the age of five, the proportion of children who were 'seldom or never jealous' rose steadily from 40 per cent of the five-year-olds to more than 50 per cent of the girls over thirteen and more than 65 per cent of the boys. At all ages girls were reported as more likely than boys to show occasional jealousy but there was no marked sex difference among the very jealous children.

Changes of Mood (Q.65)

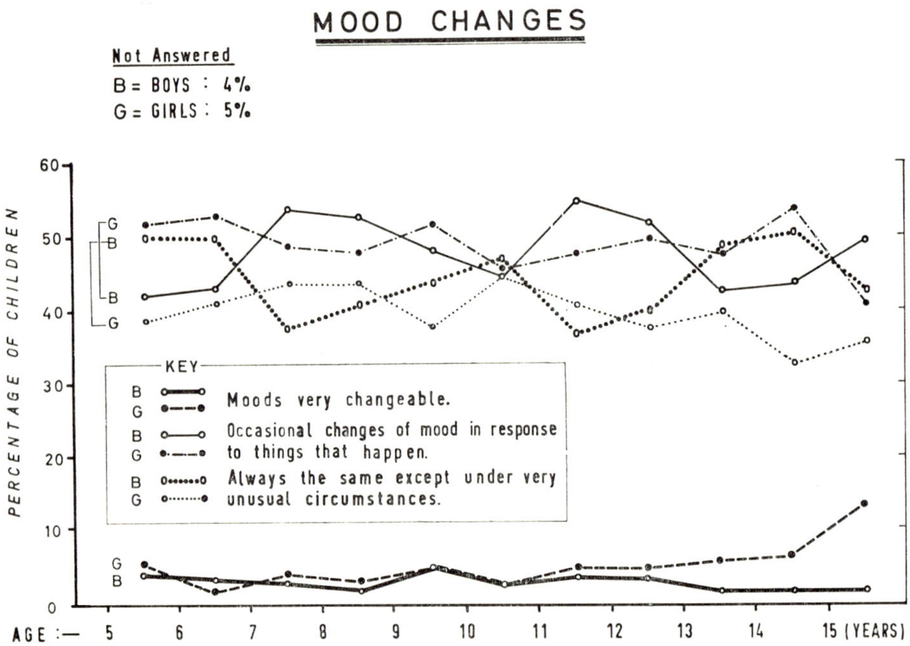

FIGURE 35

The majority of parents recorded their sons and daughters as belonging to one or other of two almost equal groups: those whose moods remained the same under most circumstances and those whose changes of mood were seen as a reasonable response to their experiences. A small minority of 4 per cent with 'very changeable' moods were reported consistently at each age up to adolescence when there was an increase among the girls and a decline among the boys. These figures were balanced by changes in the curve for placid children rather than in the intermediate category.

Worrying (Q.56)

Figure 36 shows that the proportion of children who worried 'occasionally' rose from 40 per cent among five- to six-year-olds to 70 per cent in early adolescence. Only a minority of 5 per cent in each sex, however, were described as 'often seems worried' and the numbers in this category showed no consistent relation to age. The boys were a little more likely to be regarded as 'carefree', girls to be recorded as worrying occasionally.

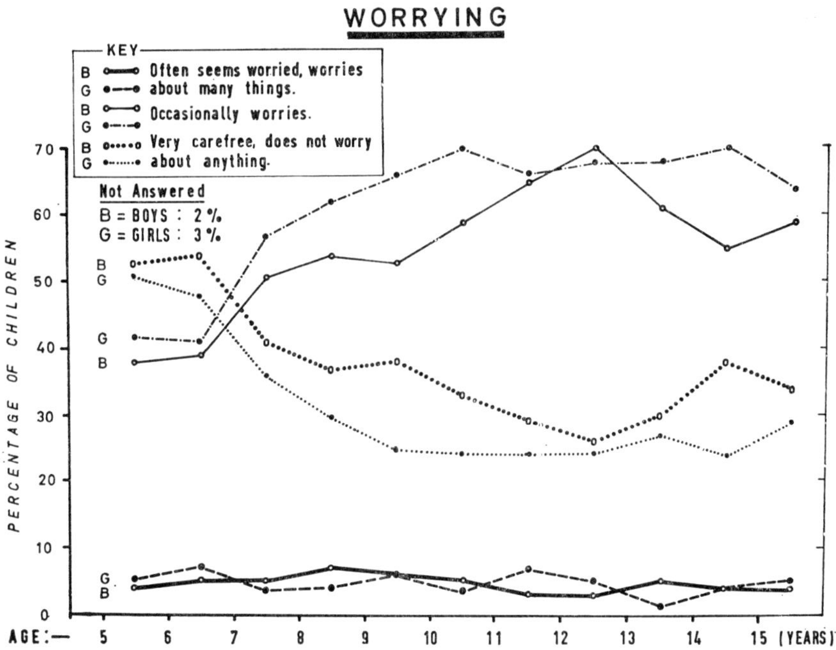

FIGURE 36

Withdrawn behaviour (Q.61)

Fewer than 3 per cent of our sample were said to be frequently withdrawn into themselves and 'out of touch with other people'. Such behaviour showed no association with age or sex. A further 35 per cent were described as 'occasionally lost in a dream world' and this category increased among girls in their teens though not among boys whose peak was at eight to nine years. Griffiths (1952) found that parents' reports showed boys to be most withdrawn between the ages of nine and eleven, whereas girls showed a steady decrease in prevalence with age.

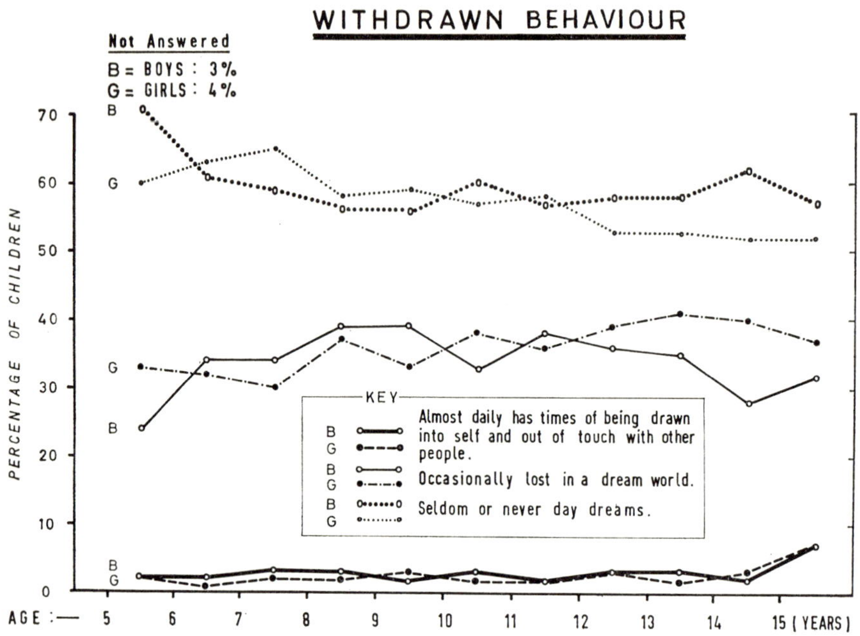

FIGURE 37

The assessment of deviance

In the preceeding analysis we have considered each type of behaviour separately. In addition, however, it was important for further analysis and research that we should have some method of grading the children in terms of the deviance of their behaviour from normality.

Table 6 shows the proportion of children at each year of age from five to fifteen who were recorded as exhibiting each of the triple-choice items of behaviour at extreme intensity. In most cases, fewer than 10 per cent of children manifested such extreme behaviour. In other instances, e.g. restlessness, food fads and reading difficulties among boys, the proportions were much higher and, on a statistical rather than a clinical basis, such behaviour could scarcely be considered abnormal.

For operational purposes we decided to make our cut-off point at the 10 per cent level. Accordingly, any type of behaviour which was recorded as occurring among 10 per cent or fewer of boys or girls, considered separately, at each year of age was assessed as deviant for children of that age and sex. Further, we decided that this criterion should apply to

TABLE 6. *Percentages of children recorded as showing 'extreme' types of behaviour at each age from five to fifteen*

GIRLS	5 *years*	6 *years*	7 *years*	8 *years*	9 *years*	10 *years*	11 *years*	12 *years*	13 *years*	14 *years*	15 *years*
Very destructive	2	—	1	—	*	*	—	*	—	1	—
Fear of animals	5	5	3	3	3	1	2	2	1	1	7
Fear of strangers	1	*	2	2	*	2	1	1	1	2	—
Fear of the dark	11	5	8	7	8	8	6	5	4	5	4
Lying	2	2	1	1	3	1	3	1	1	3	2
Dislike of school	1	3	2	4	3	2	3	3	5	7	4
Stealing	1	—	—	—	*	—	—	*	—	1	—
Irritability	10	9	9	10	12	10	12	10	11	16	11
Food fads	20	19	20	22	21	23	17	17	15	17	9
Fear of other children	—	*	1	1	*	1	*	1	*	1	—
Always hungry	5	6	6	10	9	10	10	13	15	11	16
Small appetite	21	17	21	18	13	12	12	8	7	8	5
Worrying	5	7	4	4	6	4	7	5	1	4	5
Whining	7	5	5	3	6	2	5	4	3	5	—
Restlessness	20	16	20	16	13	13	13	11	11	10	4
Underactivity	—	2	1	1	2	3	3	4	7	7	5
Jealousy	8	4	5	5	6	3	4	3	3	6	4
Wandering	*	*	—	1	1	*	1	2	1	2	4
Withdrawn	2	1	2	2	3	2	2	3	2	3	7
{ Disobedient	10	10	8	8	11	7	10	10	12	14	14
{ Always obeys	8	7	7	9	9	8	14	11	12	10	12
Truanting—at all	*	1	1	*	1	*	*	1	1	3	4
Tic	1	—	1	1	1	*	—	*	—	1	—
Mood change	5	2	4	3	5	3	5	5	7	7	14
Reading difficulty	5	7	14	14	10	13	10	11	5	7	4

BOYS	5 *years*	6 *years*	7 *years*	8 *years*	9 *years*	10 *years*	11 *years*	12 *years*	13 *years*	14 *years*	15 *years*
Very destructive	3	2	2	—	2	1	1	1	2	1	2
Fear of animals	3	3	2	1	1	2	2	1	1	1	—
Fear of strangers	2	1	1	1	—	*	*	1	2	*	4
Fear of the dark	9	6	8	8	10	7	6	5	2	2	2
Lying	5	3	5	2	3	3	3	5	4	2	2
Dislike of school	4	5	5	3	5	5	5	6	7	10	4
Stealing	—	1	1	1	1	*	1	1	2	1	—
Irritability	10	7	13	11	12	14	11	14	11	9	16
Food fads	19	20	22	22	22	18	23	19	17	17	16
Fear of other children	1	*	—	—	*	1	1	1	1	*	—
Always hungry	11	10	10	14	16	13	16	19	15	23	39
Small appetite	11	13	17	14	11	10	13	9	7	5	—
Worrying	4	5	5	7	6	5	3	3	5	4	5
Complaining	7	6	8	5	4	3	4	4	3	2	2
Restlessness	23	19	25	21	22	19	20	18	15	17	20
Underactivity	1	2	1	1	1	2	2	4	3	6	2
Jealousy	6	2	4	4	4	5	3	4	2	3	2
Wandering	3	1	2	3	3	3	3	4	4	8	2
Withdrawn	2	2	4	3	3	3	2	3	3	2	7
{ Disobedient	17	11	14	12	12	13	13	14	11	12	9
{ Always obeys	8	7	7	8	7	6	7	7	9	9	16
Truanting—at all	1	—	1	—	*	2	—	2	1	4	16
Tics	*	1	1	2	1	2	1	2	2	1	2
Mood changes	4	3	3	2	5	3	4	4	2	2	2
Reading difficulty	7	18	21	27	25	17	21	22	13	13	9

Note: * = *less than 0·5 per cent.*

behaviour at either end of the scale: as a result 'always obeys', for example, was classed as deviant behaviour for boys at nearly all ages and for girls under the age of eleven. The items which recorded behaviour in terms of frequency rather than intensity, e.g. bed-wetting, nail-biting, temper tantrums, were assessed in the same way: table 7 shows, for instance, that although reported daily crying would be deviant at any age, crying once a week or more often would not be considered deviant in children under the age of eleven.

TABLE 7. *Frequency of crying considered 'deviant' in children of different ages*

Behaviour	*Ages at which the behaviour occurred in 10 per cent or fewer of the children*	
	Boys (years)	*Girls* (years)
Crying every day or nearly every day	5–15	5–15
Crying at least two to three times a week	8–15	10–15
Crying at least once a week	11–15	11–15
Crying at least once in two weeks	12–15	12–15
Crying at least once a month	13–15	14–15
Crying at least once in two or three months	13–15	Never

Our decision to draw the line at 10 per cent was necessarily an arbitrary one. If we had adopted a 5 per cent cut-off point, fewer items would have been considered deviant though, as table 6 shows, the difference would have been surprisingly small. Had we widened our boundaries and used a 15 or 20 per cent criterion, our definition would have been in danger of becoming too wide since it would have included such categories as 'placid' boys. In practice the choice of this criterion entailed a cut-off point of 4 deviant items for the survey group as a whole (see Chapter 7).

Each child received one point towards his total deviance score for each item recorded on his questionnaire which was deviant for one of his age and sex. The distribution of total deviance scores in the sample is shown in table 8 and it is these scores which are used in later analyses, e.g. in the next chapter where the children's total deviance scores are related to some of their social characteristics and personal experiences.

TABLE 8. *Total deviance scores of children in the sample by sex*

Total deviance score	*Boys*		*Girls*	
	No.	%	*No.*	%
Nil	1224	39·3	1283	42·1
1	841	27·0	787	25·8
2	467	15·0	406	13·3
3	250	8·0	220	7·2
4	136	4·4	131	4·3
5	90	2·9	76	2·5
6	41	1·3	43	1·4
7	27		39	
8	12		19	
9	10	2·1	17	3·3
10	10		9	
11 or more	7		15	

INTER-RELATIONS BETWEEN DIFFERENT TYPES OF BEHAVIOUR

Ideally, we should have liked to describe not only the distribution of the various individual types of behaviour but also the ways in which various items of behaviour clustered together. The statistical techniques which we used in our attempts to study such behavioural patterns are summarised in Appendix 1.

Chapter Five

Social class, family size and position, health and separation experiences

In Chapter Four we considered the ways in which recorded behaviour was related to age and sex. In this chapter we examine the associations between deviant behaviour and some of the reported influences and experiences to which the children had been exposed.

Social class

The social class of the family was assessed by classifying the father's job

TABLE 9. *Association between the child's total deviance score and the father's occupational status*

	Father's occupational status group (Hall-Jones)	*Percentage of children with total deviance score of*					
		0	1	2	3	4–6	7+
1.	Professional and high administrative (N = 231)	44	29	11	6	9	1
2.	Managerial and executive (N = 371)	41	32	15	4	7	1
3.	Inspectional, supervisory and other non-manual (higher grade) (N = 655)	40	27	15	8	8	2
4.	Inspectional, supervisory and other non-manual (lower grade) (N = 547)	40	28	14	8	8	3
5a.	Routine non-manual (N = 320)	39	28	15	7	10	1
	TOTAL NON-MANUAL (N = 2124)	40	29	14	7	8	2
5b.	Skilled manual (N = 2108)	42	26	14	7	8	3
6.	Semi-skilled manual (N = 1320)	39	25	15	8	9	3
7.	Routine manual (N = 284)	39	22	14	11	10	4
	TOTAL MANUAL (N = 3712)	41	25	15	8	8	3
	Unemployed, disabled, dead (N = 106)	33	25	13	5	10	6

on the Hall-Jones scale of occupational prestige (Hall and Jones 1950). Occupation is correlated with other aspects of total socio-economic status, e.g. educational standard, income, style of life, and is therefore usually acceptable as a reasonably effective, though necessarily crude, index of social status.

Table 9 relates the child's 'total deviance score' (see page 78) to his father's type of job; it shows how little variation there was between the different status groups. In each group, approximately the same proportion of mothers were recording their children as being free of deviant items or as having exhibited four or more of such items.

Ordinal position and family size

In the popular lore of child-rearing, behaviour is often related to family composition. Thus, it has been suggested that an only child is likely to be less well adjusted because he is 'spoilt' or 'gets things too much his own way'. On the other hand, children in large families are said not to get enough love and attention from their parents. Eldest children may be subjected to parental inexperience and also feel 'pushed out' by the next arrival; youngest children may suffer at the hands of their older brothers and sisters. It is not difficult to think of good reasons why a child in any ordinal position, and in families of whatever size, might be maladjusted.

TABLE 10. *Total deviance score by position in the family*

Position in family	Percentage of children with a total deviance score of					
	0	1	2	3	4–6	7+
Only child (N = 692)	47	27	14	4	6	2
Youngest child (N = 1930)	45	26	13	8	7	1
Middle child (N = 1470)	38	27	13	9	9	4
Oldest child (N = 1960)	35	27	15	9	10	4

Note; The number of cases described in this table is slightly smaller than in table 11, as some parents failed to give detailed information about family position.

Table 10 shows that only children are the least, and oldest children are the most likely to be reported as exhibiting any deviant items of behaviour. Indeed, it appears that the presence of younger brothers and sisters is connected with a high total deviance score: the proportion of children with four or more deviant items reported is about 75 per cent

TABLE 11. *Total deviance score by size of family*

Number of siblings		Percentage of children with a total deviance score of					
		0	1	2	3	4–6	7+
None, only child	(N = 692)	47	27	14	4	6	2
1	(N = 2319)	43	26	14	7	8	2
2–3	(N = 2398)	38	27	15	8	9	3
4–5	(N = 541)	36	28	14	7	10	5
6 or more	(N = 203)	45	26	10	4	9	5

higher in the category of middle and oldest children than among those without younger siblings ($P<0{\cdot}001$).

The magnitude of the total deviance score also bears some relationship to the size of the family. Thus table 11 shows that the proportion of children with no recorded deviant items falls, and the proportion of those with a total score of four or more rises, with increasing family size up to a total of six children. In the largest families, i.e. among those children who have six or more brothers and sisters, there is again a rise in the proportion of children without deviant behaviour.

In view of the close link between family size and ordinal position the data about them can usefully be analysed together.

TABLE 12. *Percentage of children with a total deviance score of four or more by family size and position**

Family position	Family size: 2 children	3–4 children	5 or more children
Eldest	12%	13%	27%
Middle	—	13%	13%
Youngest	7%	9%	7%

* *Only children are not included in this table.*

Table 12 shows that the most deviance-prone group are the eldest children who have four or more younger brothers or sisters: 27 per cent of this group of children were recorded as manifesting four or more deviant items of behaviour compared with 12 per cent of the elder children in two-child families and only 7 per cent of the youngest children in large families.

Further analysis showed that neither the sex of the child's siblings nor the presence, nor absence, of siblings of the same sex as the individual child affected the total deviance score. However, there was some evidence to suggest that age might be relevant, particularly among the girls: girls under the age of eleven who were the eldest of their family had significantly higher deviance scores than their counterparts aged eleven or older ($P<0.05$), but among the boys the difference was smaller and not significant.

Physical health

The most commonly recorded complaints were of 'frequent colds', particularly among the younger* children in the sample; travel-sickness, most marked among the girls; and rashes and 'other skin troubles'.

TABLE 13. *Frequency of health problems as reported by the child's mother*

	Boys:		*Girls:*	
Age:	5–10 *years* (N = 1876) (%)	11–15 *years* (N = 1239) (%)	5–10 *years* (N = 1772) (%)	11–15 *years* (N = 1273) (%)
Current;				
Wears glasses always	3	5	2	4
Wears glasses sometimes	3	7	4	11
Is having treatment for eyes at clinic or hospital	3	3	3	3
Has had persistent ear-ache or running ear during the last twelve months	4	1	5	2
Seems to have difficulty in hearing sometimes	6	3	6	3
Has a hearing aid	—	—	—	—
Suffers from sick headaches	3	6	3	8
Gets travel sick in car, bus or train	16	17	25	28
Has frequent colds or sore throats	16	10	19	13
Has a persistent and troublesome cough	5	3	5	2
Is overweight	4	6	5	8
Is underweight	6	5	5	5
Has fainted more than twice in life	1	2	1	5
Has suffered from a rash or other skin trouble which lasted for two weeks or longer	11	10	10	11
Has to wear special support for bone or muscle disorder (for instance, iron on leg, built up shoe, etc.)	2	1	1	1
Has to wear brace on teeth	1	4	2	7
Has a stammer	2	2	1	1

* We have here adopted the convention of referring to the under-elevens as the 'younger' boys or girls, and to the children aged eleven and over as the 'older' ones.

TABLE 13—*continued*

	Boys:		*Girls:*	
Age:	5–10 *years* (N = 1876) (%)	11–15 *years* (N = 1239) (%)	5–10 *years* (N = 1772) (%)	11–15 *years* (N – 1273) (%)
Past or chronic; ('Has a doctor ever said that this child suffered from . . .')				
Any disease or disorder of the bones (not a broken bone)	1	1	1	1
Any disease or disorder affecting muscles	1	1	1	1
Heart trouble	1	—	1	1
Eczema	5	3	4	3
Asthma	4	3	2	2
Tuberculosis	—	—	—	—
Any chronic lung trouble (such as chronic bronchitis)	3	2	3	3
St Vitus Dance	—	—	—	—
Meningitis (Brain fever)	—	1	1	—
Migraine	1	2	—	2
Cerebral palsy ('spastic')	—	—	—	—
Fits or convulsions	1	1	1	1
Diabetes	—	—	—	—
Rheumatic fever	—	—	—	—
Hare-lip or cleft palate	—	—	—	—
Any disorder of the glands (*not* just swollen neck glands)	1	1	1	1
Hay fever and other allergies	1	1	—	1
Any other physical handicap or *chronic* illness	2	2	1	1

Very few children were said to have experienced serious illness in the past and very few to have suffered from any chronic or recurrent handicap apart from asthma, eczema or 'chronic lung trouble'. This made it impossible to relate deviant behaviour to the child's experience of a particular illness such as meningitis or diabetes. It was possible, however, to group the children according to the severity of their illnesses so as to carry out some analysis of the relation between physical health and deviant behaviour. This was done in the following way:

GROUP 1. children with *major* physical disabilities or illnesses, such as rheumatic fever, spasticity, diseases of the bones or muscles, heart trouble, etc. These totalled 478 cases, some of whom also had various minor disabilities or psychosomatic ailments.

GROUP 2. children with *minor* physical disabilities, such as persistent coughs or earache, wearing glasses or a brace on their teeth, being overweight, etc., but with no major disabilities (3 155).

GROUP 3. children with so-called *psychosomatic* complaints, chiefly 'sick headaches', but also eczema and asthma, who were not already included in groups 1 or 2 (117 children).

GROUP 4. a 'healthy' group of 2460 children with no reported physical or psychosomatic disorders.

We examined first the distribution of the most deviant children by considering the proportion of children in each group who had a total deviance score of four or more. As table 14 shows, such children were

TABLE 14. *Number of children with various types of physical disorder showing the percentage scoring four or more deviant items of behaviour*

	Major physical disorder (Group 1)	*Minor physical disorder* (Group 2)	*Psychosomatic disorder* (Group 3)	*No disability* (Group 4)
Girls aged 5–10 years	130	940	18	682
Girls aged 11–15 years	97	713	27	407
Boys aged 5–10 years	148	904	37	817
Boys aged 11–15 years	103	598	35	554
All children	478	3155	117	2460
Percentage of the total having a total deviance score of four or more	22%	16%	10%	7%

found significantly ($P<0{\cdot}001$) more often in the groups of children with some degree of health problem than in the 'healthy' group. It is also noticeable that the group of children with major disabilities or a history of serious illness contained a greater proportion of high deviance scores than did the group with only minor disorders. Children with psychosomatic ailments but no other recorded health problems did not appear to differ markedly from the 'healthy' group in respect of deviance. The children in group 3, however, are not neccessarily representative of all those with psychosomatic ailments. In table 15 (page 86) we have compared the total deviance scores of the children with only psychosomatic disorders (group 3) with the scores of those sub-groups of children recorded as suffering from psychosomatic illness as well as from some major or minor disorder. The figures show clearly that the deviance score in mixed cases is related to the degree of severity of the other category of disorder ($P<0{\cdot}01$) rather than to the tendency to suffer from psychosomatic illness. This does not, however, signify that the experience of a serious illness must in itself lead to deviant conduct since the children in this category had also been in hospital more often and for longer periods than the others. They were also about twice as likely as the children with recorded minor disorders to have undergone surgery while in hospital.

TABLE 15. *Percentage of children with psychosomatic illnesses, with and without other physical disorders, who had total deviance scores of four or more*

	N	*Percentage scoring 4 or more deviant items*
Children with psychosomatic illness only	117	10
Psychosomatic illness and minor physical disorders	89	18
Psychosomatic illness and major physical disorders	475	28

When recorded physical disorders were related to individual types of behaviour, the children who had experienced severe disorders were reported significantly more often than those with minor disorders to cry, to be irritable, to have tantrums and to quarrel with other children. Comparative differences were recorded concerning restlessness, both in their waking hours and in their sleep, but not in respect of anxiety, fear or withdrawn behaviour.

Reactions to menstruation

The mothers of girls of all ages in our sample were asked whether their daughters had started to menstruate and, if so, at what age. Five categories were also asked about the girl's reaction to her period: 1. worries about it; 2. feels sick; 3. complains of pains; 4. has to stay away from school or go to bed; 5. usually has no trouble or worry at all. The answers to these questions were then related to one another, to the child's age at the time of the survey, and to the total deviance score.

There were altogether 565 girls in our sample who were recorded as having started menstruation at the time of our survey. Some two-thirds of them were said not to experience any worries or discomforts at all during their periods; those who were so troubled complained about pains but only rarely did they feel sick or have to stay away from school.

No significant relation was found between earlier age of onset and the number of complaints recorded. Certainly there was no evidence to suggest that girls with an early menarche were likely to find it more troublesome; if anything, there was a slight trend in the reverse direction.

The age of onset of menstruation was also tabulated against the total deviance score for each girl but no significant association was found. When, however, reported menstrual discomfort was related to the total deviance score it emerged that 22 per cent of girls who suffered in this way had scored four or more items, whereas this was only true of 14 per cent of those said to experience 'no worry or trouble at all' ($P<0{\cdot}01$). It was confirmed that this was not due to the contribution of 'pains in stomach' to the total deviance score. Menstrual discomfort may, then, be connected with a general pattern of deviance. On the other hand it may indicate a lower standard of health since the girls who were recorded as suffering from a major physical disorder (see page 84) were more likely to have been recorded as suffering from painful periods than were other girls ($P<0{\cdot}05$).

Admission to hospital

In table 16 (page 88) we see the detailed distribution of hospital admissions by frequency, duration and cause. While the majority of children had never been admitted to hospital, the proportion of in-patients inevitably increased with age. Among the children who were admitted to hospital, most had only been in on one occasion and had only stayed for a relatively short time: nearly a quarter of the children had been discharged within three days. About three-quarters of the children underwent surgery, mainly removal of tonsils and adenoids. Gastro-intestinal disorders were the next most frequent cause of admission, followed by orthopaedic conditions and accidents.

Clearly, the children had been admitted to and discharged from hospital at varying times before our survey was conducted. This made it impossible to estimate accurately the immediate effects on a child's behaviour of his stay in hospital. However, the mother was asked to record her memory of the circumstances. The results are summarised in table 17 on page 89 which indicates that the longer the time spent by the child in hospital, the more likely was he or she to be recorded as having displayed behaviour difficulties on returning home. Also more than four-fifths of the children who had been in hospital were not reported as having shown any adverse effects on their return home. Some, indeed,

TABLE 16. *Hospital in-patient treatment*

	Boys 5–10 years (%)	*Boys* 11–15 years (%)	*Girls* 5–10 years (%)	*Girls* 11–15 years (%)
a. *Number of admissions*	(N = 1876)	(N = 1239)	(N = 1772)	(N = 1273)
None	60	53	67	54
One admission	31	35	28	34
Two admissions	6	8	4	8
Three admissions	2	2	1	2
Four admissions	—	1	—	1
More than four admissions	—	—	—	1
b. *Accumulated duration of stay**†	(N = 741)	(N = 581)	(N = 586)	(N = 568)
Up to 3 days	25	18	27	21
4 days to 6 days inclusive	19	19	21	18
7 days to 13 days inclusive	25	27	24	23
14 days to 20 days inclusive	10	11	8	13
21 days up to 1 month	7	10	9	10
1 month up to 3 months	10	11	9	10
3 months up to 6 months	2	2	2	2
6 months or longer	2	2	1	1
c. *Reasons for admission**‡	(N = 741)	(N = 581)	(N = 586)	(N = 568)
Neuro-psychiatric (tics, epilepsy, meningitis, encephalitis etc.)	2	2	3	3
Allergic diseases (e.g. asthma)	1	1	1	1
Ear, nose and throat disorders	58	64	61	67
Congenital disorders (squint, harelip, cleft palate, removal of extra toes, treatment for bone distortion, cosmetic or plastic surgery)	7	5	8	5
Gastro-intestinal disorders	15	15	11	13
Orthopaedic disorders, and accidents (broken bones, scalds, shock or observation after accidents, arrow in eye, half drowned, car accidents, swallowing unsuitable objects, etc.)	12	14	10	9
Cardiovascular and respiratory disorders	6	5	5	6
Infectious diseases, fevers, etc.	5	5	4	6
Dermatological disorders	2	1	1	—
Miscellaneous (e.g. diabetes)	13	11	7	9
Surgical intervention of any kind	73	77	71	77

* *In sections b) and c) of the table the percentages have been calculated as proportions of the number of children who have been admitted to hospital, and not of the total sample.*

† *The accumulated duration of stay is the total time a child has spent in hospital when all his admissions are combined.*

‡ *Since these categories are not mutually exclusive, any child can be recorded as being admitted to hospital for more than one reason, particularly if he has been admitted more than once.*

were said to have improved in that they were, for example, eating better or had stopped thumb-sucking. It is possible that the relatively small number of children reported to have experienced behaviour disturbance is attributable to the retrospective nature of the data, which depends on the

TABLE 17. *Proportion of children reported by their parents to show behaviour problems on return home from hospital, related to cumulative length of stay in hospital (all ages, both sexes)*

Length of hospital stay	*Number of cases*	*Percentage showing behaviour problems*
Up to 3 days	569	9
4–6 days	492	11
7–13 days	625	12
14–30 days	497	13
1–3 months	259	21
Over 3 months	87	22

mother's accurate recall of past events. On the other hand, a stay in hospital is usually a dramatic event in the life of both the child and his mother so that the attendant circumstances are likely to be remembered.

Table 18 shows the distribution of total deviance scores among children who had been in hospital for differing periods of time and, as can be seen, there appears to be little association between the two variables. It must be noted, however, that table 18 describes the reported state at the date of our survey of children who had been admitted to hospital at all ages from immediately after birth until the age of fifteen; furthermore, the

TABLE 18. *Distribution of total deviance scores by age at survey and cumulative duration of hospital in-patient treatment*

Cumulative duration of hospital in-patient treatment	*Percentage of children aged 5–10 years with total deviance score of*						*Total no. of children aged 5-10 years*	*Percentage of children aged 11-15 years with total deviance score of*						*Total no. of children aged 11-15 years*
	0	1	2	3	4-6	7+		0	1	2	3	4-6	7+	
None	42	27	14	7	8	2	2321	46	25	13	6	7	2	1363
Less than 7 days	36	26	18	9	9	2	602	44	24	14	7	8	3	440
7-13 days	33	27	14	11	11	4	326	37	30	10	9	10	4	285
2 weeks-1 month	35	23	15	10	11	6	225	42	23	13	8	10	4	248
1-3 months	33	28	19	7	10	2	127	31	31	11	9	10	7	118
3 months or longer	27	39	7	12	5	10	41	34	27	21	7	10	—	29

interval which had elapsed between discharge from hospital and our investigation was subject to considerable variation from one child to another. While, therefore, our figures cannot support any suggestion that hospital admission has lasting adverse effects on children in general, neither can they be taken as reputing any suggestions that hospitalisation may have a deleterious effect on children at particular stages of their development.

Separation experiences

The various theories concerning the effects of separation (Yarrow 1961) suggest that it is a complex concept which incorporates several factors, including the length of separation; the age or developmental stage at which it occurs; the reason for separation, e.g. because of the child's illness, the break-up of the home, the birth of a new baby, etc; the form taken by the separation, e.g. whether the child goes to hospital, stays with relatives, or goes to a children's home; the frequency with which separation takes place; and the extent to which the child has expressed distress during the separation or immediately after reunion with the parents. While some information was available on all these issues, we did not have a sufficient number of cases of separation to allow us to explore all possible combinations.

The questionnaire included a number of items concerning separation from parents experienced by the child. In addition to admissions to hospital, which we have already mentioned in this chapter, data were collected about any other occasions on which the child had been away from home, without his parents, for more than a month. We also inquired whether either parent had been away from home for any reason for at least a month since the child's birth and whether the mother worked outside the home. These data are not, of course, as comprehensive as would be desirable for a study specifically devoted to separation and its effects. They suffer from the defects of all retrospective studies, including the dangers of inaccurate recall by the parents, the lack of information about the child's behaviour before any separation took place and about contaminating influences bearing on the child between the separation experience and the time of the survey. Moreover the variety of some causes of separation such as death of a parent and the lack of detail in some answers make a rigorous analysis impossible. Nevertheless, since the subject is an important and controversial one, we have included some discussion of the association between deviance and separation.

Nearly a quarter of the children (23 per cent) had experienced separation from at least one parent because of that parent's absence from home for a period of a month or longer. The separation involved only the father in the majority of cases (13 per cent of the sample) but the mothers of 9 per cent of the children had been away for at least a month and 2 per cent of children had experienced such separation from both parents, though not necessarily at the same time.

TABLE 19. *Total deviance score by parental absence*

	Younger boys	*Older boys*	*Younger girls*	*Older girls*	*All*
N =	1869	1236	1770	1273	
Neither away	9%	11%	11%	15%	11%
Father away	11%	12%	12%	23%	14%
Mother away	19%	13%	15%	27%	18%
Both away (at different times)	33%	24%	7%	34%	25%

Entries represent the number of children with a total deviance score of four or more items, calculated as a percentage of the total number of children in the category indicated.

Table 19 shows the relation between parents' absence from home and a total deviance score of at least four items. Absence of both parents, even though at different times, was associated with the highest proportion of 'deviant' children; this association was less marked with a recorded absence of the mother only, and still less with that of the father alone. The pattern was consistent and statistically significant for three out of the four age/sex groups; the younger girls constituted the only exception.

With regard to the children's own absences from home, 6 per cent of the younger age group in both sexes and 8 per cent of the older children were reported to have been away for at least one period of a month or more apart from any admissions to hospital. Unfortunately it was not possible to carry out a more detailed analysis of such absence because of the lack of sufficient information about the child's age when separation took place and where each child spent this period, e.g. with relatives or with strangers.

Reported hospital admissions, as we have already shown in table 16, were more common: between 12 and 15 per cent of children were said to have been in-patients for at least four weeks, though this period might have been spread over several admissions.

The analysis so far has treated the various types of separation as though they were independent. Often, however, this was not the case: a child might, for example, have had to stay with relatives because the mother was away in hospital. Other children might have experienced various categories of separation at different times.

TABLE 20. *Number of children with different combinations of reported separation experiences*

		Number of children			
		Boys (aged 5–10)	*Boys* (aged 11–15)	*Girls* (aged 5–10)	*Girls* (aged 11–15)
Mother away					
*Child away**					
Hospital stay†	(Long)	11	14	12	11
	(Short)	27	14	7	19
	(None)	29	15	38	23
*Child not away**					
Hospital stay†	(Long)	19	36	17	26
	(Short)	30	39	41	33
	(None)	67	50	62	61
Mother not away					
*Child away**					
Hospital stay†	(Long)	7	15	4	12
	(Short)	13	16	10	18
	(None)	31	24	27	25
*Child not away**					
Hospital stay†	(Long)	186	159	130	146
	(Short)	438	312	351	278
	(None)	997	548	1 001	541

* *This refers to any period of at least a month's absence from home, apart from time spent in hospital.*

† *A 'long hospital stay' is defined as one lasting at least two weeks; a 'short hospital stay' is one of less than two weeks.*

These cases are analysed in table 20 on a basis of three types of separation, namely *a*) whether or not the mother had been away from home for any period lasting at least a month; *b*) whether or not the child had been absent from home for a period of a month or more, apart from any admissions to hospital; and *c*) whether the child had been in hospital for at least two weeks, for less than two weeks, or not at all.

The findings demonstrate that many of the children were recorded in more than one category. For instance, among the children whose mothers had been away from home for at least a month, two-thirds had also been in hospital themselves and one in five had not only been in hospital but had also been living away from home for at least a month for some other reason.

TABLE 21. *Reported separation and total deviance score: percentage of the children in each cell with 4 + deviant items*

	Separation experience				
	Mother away		*Mother not away*		
	Child away	*Child not away*	*Child away*	*Child not away*	*Total*
Hospital stay:					
Long	29%	19%	26%	13%	16%
Short	27%	15%	18%	12%	13%
None	22%	12%	21%	9%	10%
All:	18%		11%		

Table 21 relates the total deviance scores of four and more items to the various combinations of types of separation. The broad pattern is clear: all three types of separation were associated with a larger proportion of children with high deviance scores. Furthermore, this association is cumulative: the children with no separation experiences included the lowest proportion of 'deviants'; the group of children with only one period of separation contained fewer 'deviants' than the group with two periods of separation; and those children who fell into all three separation categories showed the highest proportion of 'deviants'.

It would be hazardous, on this evidence, to suggest that one type of separation rather than another is linked with a high total deviance score. The association is a complex one and requires more detailed examination than was possible with the data at our disposal. Only further research will show, for instance, to what extent separation experiences merely accentuate a pre-existing condition, and in what ways a variety of intervening variables can sharpen or modify this pattern of association.

A special study was made of a small group of forty-nine children in our sample who had experienced exceptional numbers, varieties and degrees of separation. A closer examination of the data indicated their complexity with regard to the numerous additional influences which were at work within the family, and which may have influenced both the impact of the various separation experiences and the child's later mental health.

The following are some examples of condensed records of children who had all spent at least fourteen days in hospital at one time or another, and who had also experienced other forms of separation:

1. G., a boy aged eight, had been in hospital twice, the first time for twelve weeks at the age of five months, with whooping cough and pneumonia; the second time for a week when he was six. After the second admission the mother said that he was 'very slow to mix with people, he seemed to want to stop round me all the time'. He was in two children's homes while his mother was in hospital; for one month when he was four, and three months when he was two years old. His mother reported disobedience, headaches, stomach pains, reading difficulties. The teacher commented: 'The income at home is not used in the best way', and noted: 'Has speech difficulty, sucks finger, unco-operative in class, very quiet and withdrawn, not interested in his work.'

2. M., a boy aged eight, had been in hospital for ten days for an operation when he was four and again for ten days at the age of five because of an accident. His father and mother had both been away from home for more than a month at some time. His mother wrote: 'He was away when I went into hospital, he was away for three months in Dr Barnardo's home, as there was nobody to have them and I felt they would be safe there. He is at home now, that was four years ago.' She reported fear of the dark, excessive appetite, disobedience, crying, temper tantrums. The teacher noted: 'bites finger nails, not interested in school work', and commented: 'large family—eight children. The father died about four years ago, when the youngest child was a baby. The mother remarried almost immediately. She works in a transport cafe but there always seems to be a shortage of money, difficulty in getting dinner-money, never the odd copper to spend on sweets, no money for school outings, etc. . . . The children are always poorly clad, in need of hair cut and have little or no mending done to their clothes.'

3. T., a boy aged eleven, had been in hospital for ten months at the age of three, suffering from tuberculosis. 'When T. had T.B. I had it also,' his mother wrote. 'He was sent home but I had to stay and undergo an operation so my mother cared for him for five months, but they were very attached to each other. I was then home and able to care for him myself.' The mother reported that T. displayed irritability, excessive appetite, constipation, restless sleep, nail-biting. He was also overweight and had an orthopaedic disorder. At school he was said to be very quiet and withdrawn. 'I would say his lethargy is due to his over-size,' his teacher wrote.

4. M., a boy aged fourteen, was in hospital for four weeks at the age of three with suspected tuberculosis of the hip, for three weeks at the age of nine, and again for one week at the age of eleven for the same complaint. In connection with the first illness the mother reported that 'we were not allowed to visit M. and when he returned home he was very black round the eyes, was very nervy and a different child. When he was in hospital later I was allowed to stay nights at first and visit every day and he was happy.' The mother has been away from home herself on one occasion. When the child 'lived with friends and aunts for six months while I was in (a mental hospital). I am sorry to say that (the child) has a very unhappy background and is being rather difficult at the present time.' She reported fear of the dark, nightmares, restless sleep, nail-biting, reading difficulties.

5. A., a girl aged fourteen, who had been in hospital for three weeks at the age of three with scarlet fever and for one week at the age of ten to have her tonsils out. The mother wrote: 'She lived with an aunt in the country for eighteen months when I first began working in London. It took eighteen months for me to find a place suitable for her to live in. I visited her at least once a month and sometimes more. . . . A shy and lonely child. She is afraid to ask her teachers anything and often gives an opposite impression. She has no interest in clothes and the usual things a girl of fourteen would be interested in. She is very withdrawn and finds it difficult to make friends. Our relationship, however, is excellent.' She reported fear of the dark and nail-biting. The girl's parents had been recently divorced. The school found her very quiet and withdrawn.

6. B., a girl aged fourteen, had been in hospital for four months with a broken leg and hip at the age of six and 'was in twice before with bronchial pneumonia and chicken-pox'. The mother reported destructiveness, lying, dislike of school, irritability, food fads, whining, restlessness, jealousy, disobedience, crying, sulking, temper tantrums, nail-biting, quarrelling. She also said that the girl 'swears at me when she can't have her own way and accuses me of everything. I wish she was away as she causes a lot of trouble when she is at home.' The girl had stayed at a residential special school. The teacher wrote that she was scholastically 'very, very weak, seems to have low intelligence. Family seems shiftless and to have very little control over B.'

It is obvious from a perusal of such cases that they make up a heterogeneous group. Some admissions to hospital were attributable to illness, others to accidents; and these events had taken place at varying periods of time in the past. Hospital visiting and pre-existing family circumstances may have influenced the eventual outcome, and the histories included instances of mothers being seriously ill, fathers dying and mothers re-marrying, divorce and migration. There was also a group of families which seemed somewhat generally unstable, so that the child's behaviour might have been due to many kinds of stresses, in addition to the various separations. In such cases the implications of separation are clearly difficult to distinguish from the child's background and family history.

Chapter Six

The child at school

As we have already shown (in Chapter 2) it was regarded as important to obtain information about the child at school as well as at home. Questionnaires (see Appendix 3) were, therefore, presented to teachers as well as parents (see Chapter 3); they were completed and returned by the schools in 97 per cent of cases. The majority (68 per cent) of the children were still of primary school age; among those who had reached secondary school 28 per cent attended grammar or technical schools, 72 per cent were at secondary modern schools. Only 1 per cent of the children were at special schools for the physically or mentally handicapped.

Attainment

For the reasons already discussed in Chapter 2 (page 27) we decided to limit our classification of attainment to three broad categories: the teacher was asked to assess the child as 'average', 'above average' or 'below average' compared with others of the same age attending the same type of school. This procedure, though open to the disadvantage that the teacher's assessment may be subject to a halo effect or some other forms of bias, at least provided an indication of the child's success in the environment of his particular type of school. It was supplemented by a question about the child's relative success in his immediate teaching group. Clearly this could be different from the first assessment: a child at the top of the bottom stream of a large school would be below average compared with all pupils of his age at the school but yet be a success in his own classroom.

Table 22 confirms the findings of other surveys (Pidgeon 1960, Wisenthal 1965) that girls are rated higher in attainment than boys, particularly in the younger age groups. Thus, among the five- to ten-year-olds, 23 per cent of the girls were graded above average in general attainment compared with only 16 per cent of the boys. Among those over ten

TABLE 22. *Teachers' ratings of general attainment and reading ability relative to age and types of school attended*

Teacher's rating (relative to age and type of school)	*General attainment* Boys (%)	Girls (%)	*Reading ability* Boys (%)	Girls (%)
Above average	18	22	20	25
Average	45	51	42	48
Below average	34	24	28	18
Not yet learned to read	—	—	3	2
Not recorded	3	3	7	7
Total number of children	3477 (100%)	3234 (100%)	3477 (100%)	3234 (100%)

years of age the proportion of above average girls had fallen to 18 per cent and that of boys had risen to 19 per cent. The picture for children graded as above average readers was very similar. At the other end of the scale, however, there was no corresponding change since 34 per cent of boys and 24 per cent of girls were reported as below average in general attainment in both age groups. Poor readers, on the other hand, showed a more encouraging picture: among the eleven- to fifteen-year-olds 22 per cent of boys and 14 per cent of girls were below average (including non-readers) compared

TABLE 23. *Association between the child's general attainment and the occupational status of the father on the Hall-Jones Scale*

Father's occupational grouping (Hall-Jones Scale)	*Percentages of boys with fathers in each group*			*Total number of boys*	*Percentages of girls with fathers in each group*			*Total number of girls*
	Above average attainment	*Average attainment*	*Below average attainment*		*Above average attainment*	*Average attainment*	*Below average attainment*	
1, 2, 3. Professional managerial, higher grade supervisory	29	49	22	600	37	48	15	624
4, 5a. Lower grade supervisory, routine non-manual	23	48	29	424	29	52	19	402
5b. Skilled manual	17	47	36	1011	17	56	27	979
6, 7. Semi- or unskilled manual	14	44	42	800	17	48	35	639
All children	19	47	34	2832	23	53	24	2754

with 36 per cent of boys and 24 per cent of girls in the younger age groups. Here there has been an apparent improvement in reading ability in both sexes, leaving the boys at the same comparative disadvantage as before.

The general attainment level was found to be associated with the socio-economic background of the child, as assessed by the father's occupational status on the Hall-Jones scale.

Table 23 shows that, in a comparison of the extremes of the occupational ladder, the children of fathers in professional, managerial or high supervisory positions were twice as likely to be graded as above average in attainment and half as likely to be classed below average as were those children with fathers in semi-skilled or unskilled manual employment. Among both boys and girls the attainment level is clearly correlated with the level of skill and prestige involved in the father's occupational grading.

This relationship appeared to hold at all ages. Among boys aged five to ten years, 28 per cent of those whose fathers' jobs were in the highest status groups were of 'above average' attainment and 23 per cent 'below average' compared with 30 per cent and 22 per cent respectively among boys aged eleven to fifteen; 44 per cent of boys aged five to ten years with fathers in semi-skilled or unskilled jobs were graded 'below average' and

TABLE 24. *Position in class by father's occupational status*

Father's occupational class	*No. and percentage of children in each class position* 5–10 age group						11–15 age group					
	In top 25% *of class*		*In middle* 25% *of class*		*In bottom* 25% *of class*		*In top* 25% *of class*		*In middle* 25% *of class*		*In bottom* 25% *of class*	
	No.	%	*No.*	%	*No.*	%	*No.*	%	*No.*	%	*No.*	%
BOYS												
1, 2, 3. Professional, managerial and higher grade supervisory.	147	39	150	39	82	22	57	26	123	57	37	17
4, 5a. Lower supervisory and routine non-manual.	97	36	116	43	56	21	41	26	78	49	41	26
5b. Skilled manual.	151	24	287	46	192	30	123	31	193	49	80	20
6, 7. Semi- and un-skilled manual.	88	18	224	47	168	35	78	25	147	47	85	27
Significance of association	$P<0{\cdot}001$						$P<0{\cdot}05$					
GIRLS												
1, 2 : 3. Professional, managerial and higher grade supervisory.	194	52	146	39	34	9	90	36	111	45	48	19
4, 5a. Lower supervisory and routine non-manual.	87	37	112	47	37	16	63	35	83	46	36	20
5b. Skilled manual	155	28	284	50	124	22	112	27	223	53	83	20
6, 7. Semi- and un-skilled manual.	108	24	214	48	125	28	77	27	145	50	65	23
Significance of association	$P<0{\cdot}001$						$P<0{\cdot}05$: not significant					

so were 39 per cent of such boys in the eleven to fifteen years range. Similarly, among the girls 13 per cent of those with fathers in status groups 1, 2 or 3, and 31 per cent of those with semi-skilled or unskilled fathers were rated 'below average' in the younger age groups compared with 17 per cent and 29 per cent respectively among the older girls. Overall, there was no significant difference between the two age groups in either sex.

The situation was different, however, with respect to position in the classroom (see table 24). Socio-economic differences were much more marked in the primary school children where they were highly significant ($P<0{\cdot}001$); in the secondary school age groups such differences were only just significant at the 5 per cent level for boys, and non-significant for girls. This may well have been due to the increase of streaming by ability at secondary school ages. The children who were top of unstreamed primary classes came into competition only with those of approximately their own attainment level, and the same was true of children at each level of intelligence and attainment. In particular, the favourable position of children with fathers in professional and other 'high' status occupations was significantly less evident in secondary school life ($P<0{\cdot}001$ in each sex). Among the girls age differences in other occupational groups were not significant but among the boys both the children of skilled manual workers ($P<0{\cdot}05$) and those of semi-skilled and unskilled fathers ($P<0{\cdot}001$) were in a significantly more favourable position after leaving primary school.

Absence from school

Table 25 shows that absence during the previous term was highest among the youngest children in the sample, i.e. the five- and six-year-olds, whose average loss of schooling was about twice as great as that of children aged ten or eleven. This may be a reflection of the increased exposure to infection which results from the child's introduction to the wider school society (Norris 1951). In the teens there was a tendency for frequency of absence to rise again, but never to the same level as in the infant school groups.

Among the youngest age groups the child's own illness accounted for nearly all absence. Other causes became more evident among the older children but, nevertheless, illness continued to account for at least four-fifths of absence at all age levels. Absence of the child because of the illness of some other family member was recorded most often of the older children, in particular the older girls who, obviously, were able to help most in domestic crises. Thus, 7 per cent of girls aged thirteen to fifteen

TABLE 25. *Average number of half-day sessions lost through absence in previous complete term by age and sex*

Age	*Average absence (half-day sessions)*	
	Boys	*Girls*
5 years	18·9	17·2
6 years	15·5	15·8
7 years	11·8	12·9
8 years	11·1	10·2
9 years	7·9	10·2
10 years	7·7	9·0
11 years	8·0	8·8
12 years	7·7	9·2
13 years	8·3	10·4
14 years	9·7	9·6
15 years	9·5	11·9
All ages	10·4	11·1

years had missed school because of the illness of a parent or other family member compared with 3 per cent of those aged ten to twelve and 2 per cent of those under ten years. Such absence was much rarer among the boys where it applied to only 4 per cent of the fourteen- to fifteen-year-olds and to less than 2 per cent of those under fourteen.

Truancy, a relatively rare phenomenon, was, on the other hand, more characteristic of boys than of girls. Thus of the forty-nine cases reported, thirty-eight (77 per cent) were boys. The majority (68 per cent) of truants were over twelve years of age and the number of truants rose steadily throughout the teens to reach a peak at 5 per cent of fourteen-year-old boys and 9 per cent of those aged fifteen.

After entry to secondary school there was also an increased incidence in the number of odd days on which a child, apparently with parental support, did not attend school but had no valid excuse to offer for absence. For example, such absence was attributed to only 4 per cent of five- to ten-year-old boys compared with 7 per cent of those aged eleven or more. Among the girls the rate remained constant at 4 per cent at all ages except twelve, when it rose to 7 per cent, and fifteen, when 20 per cent had such absence recorded.

Behaviour

More than half of the children (55 per cent of boys, 61 per cent of girls) had no behaviour problems noted by their teachers* but boys were

* The teachers' questionnaire is shown in Appendix 3, page 220.

more likely to have had at least one item marked★ than girls ($P<0.001$).

TABLE 26. *Number and percentage of children of all ages for whom teachers underlined the behaviour mentioned*

Behaviour	*Boys* (N = 3177) *No.*	%	*Girls* (N = 3234) *No.*	%
Very restless, etc.*	342	9·8	128	4·0
Very quiet, withdrawn*	351	10·1	456	14·1
Not interested in school work*	248	7·1	135	4·2
Bites finger nails	227	6·5	231	7·1
Worries more than others	313	6·1	213	6·6
Other speech difficulty*	172	4·9	71	2·2
Aggressive to other children*	169	4·9	71	2·2
Very easily frightened	160	4·6	133	4·1
Very shy, etc.	149	4·3	153	4·7
Unco-operative in class*	138	4·0	63	1·9
Very irritable, etc.	130	3·7	99	3·1
Often tells lies*	115	3·3	51	1·6
Cries more than most children	83	2·4	70	2·2
Sucks thumb or finger	79	2·3	96	3·0
Very moody, etc.	69	2·0	58	1·8
Has stolen once†	64	1·8	31	1·0
One or more tantrums at school	62	1·8	41	1·3
Stammers*	52	1·5	17	0·5
Showed fear of entering school in current year	49	1·4	43	1·3
Noticeable twitch*	38	1·1	11	0·3
Wet or soiled self at school	33	0·9	24	0·7

* *Sex difference significant at 0·1 per cent level.*

† *Sex difference significant at 1 per cent level.*

Table 26 shows that boys were more likely than girls to have been credited with difficult behaviour in school—restlessness, lack of interest, aggressiveness, lack of co-operation in class, lying and stealing—and to have had twitches, stammers and other speech difficulties. Girls, on the other hand, were significantly more likely to have been rated as very quiet and withdrawn.

For each sex there was a tendency for the average number of items noted by teachers to fall after the age of nine, though there was a slight upward trend among the fifteen-year-olds in their last months at school. Part of the decline may have been due to individual teachers in secondary schools having had less contact with one particular group of children since they taught their speciality to many classes and did not concentrate on one form as in primary schools. Nevertheless there was also evidence of changes relating to the age of the children and some of the individual behavioural

★ As quiet and withdrawn behaviour was the only item to be recorded in more than 10 per cent of cases it was not considered appropriate to adopt a general measure of deviance in this case.

items were relatively rare outside the infant school group. Thus the five- to seven-year-olds, though only constituting about 30 per cent of the whole sample, accounted for over two-thirds of those who seemed afraid of school or who soiled or wet themselves while there, and over half of the reported cases of thumb-sucking, excessive crying and being easily frightened. Among the boys, reported anxiety at school and aggression towards other children were also at their peak among the five- to seven-year-olds and then declined; the girls showed little decrease in such behaviour before the age of twelve. On the other hand, there was a decreasing prevalence of reported speech disorders among girls after the age of seven, while for boys the rate remained constant until the age of eleven. Restlessness and shyness of other children both gradually decreased among the boys as they grew older, with the highest prevalence among five-year-olds in each case. The girls showed little variation in restlessness with age. Similarly, though shyness was most frequently noted among five- to six-year-olds, there were also subsidiary peaks at ten and fifteen, so that no consistent pattern could be observed.

Quiet or withdrawn behaviour and nail-biting were most often reported of children in the middle of their schooling, i.e. aged between nine and twelve. Irritability also showed some tendency to rise in each sex between ten and eleven and increased markedly among fifteen-year-old boys. Lack of interest in school work and poor cooperation in class were particularly characteristic of adolescence, with a peak prevalence among fourteen- and fifteen-year-olds.

The remaining types of behaviour listed on the questionnaire—tantrums, moodiness, lying, stealing, stammering and having a tic—were not related to age in either sex.

Relation of school behaviour to attainment

Table 27 (page 104) shows that behaviour problems in school were associated with poor attainment, supporting the results of previous enquiries such as those of Scott (1958b) and Chazan (1963). Over half the boys and nearly two-thirds of the girls rated by their teacher as being of below average attainment had at least one reported behaviour problem, compared with only about one in four of those rated above-average in each sex. At the other end of the scale the children with poor attainment were three times as likely to have had four or more behavioural items underlined as were those with average attainment.

TABLE 27. *General attainment level by number of problems of behaviour underlined by the child's teacher*

No. of problems underlined by teachers	Boys: Above average No.	%	Boys: Average No.	%	Boys: Below average No.	%	Girls: Above average No.	%	Girls: Average No.	%	Girls: Below average No.	%
Nil	407	72	874	62	388	38	492	75	987	64	317	45
1	103	18	318	23	285	28	121	18	340	22	202	28
2	32	6	122	9	165	16	30	5	135	9	102	14
3	18	3	40	3	83	8	9	1	55	4	42	6
4 or more	9	2	43	3	91	9	5	1	32	2	46	6
Total	569	100	1397	100	1012	100	657	100	1549	100	709	100

Boys (attainment level relative to age): By χ^2—test, $P<0{\cdot}001$

Girls (attainment level relative to age): By χ^2—test, $P<0{\cdot}001$

A comparison of the prevalence of the various types of behaviour among children rated as of above average, and below average attainment respectively, showed some variation according to age and sex. Each sex was therefore divided into *a*) a younger group aged five to ten, and *b*) an older group aged eleven to fifteen; each of the four groups was then analysed separately.

Table 28 shows that children rated as below-average in attainment tended to exhibit two types of problems in their classroom behaviour to a significantly greater extent than did average or above average children. On the one hand, they were characterized by a marked lack of interest in school work; this item was underlined for 17 per cent of the boys and 13 per cent of the girls who were below average, compared with 1 per cent of of the boys and 0·3 per cent of the girls in the above-average group and 2 per cent of children of average attainment in each sex. Possibly as a result of this lack of interest, they were also more likely to have been recorded as behaving in ways which were disturbing to classroom routine—showing lack of co-operation in class, frequent lying and restlessness (except for the older girls). On the other hand, the children rated as below average were also more likely than other children to show recessive behaviour at school: they were significantly more often described as 'easily frightened', 'quiet or withdrawn' (except the older boys), 'shy, finds it difficult to mix with other children' (boys only) and 'afraid of school' (younger age-groups only). Also associated with poor attainment were habits such as nail-biting and thumb-sucking among the younger children and speech difficulties other than stammering. Emotional reactions—moodiness, temper tantrums, crying, irritability—were not found to be associated with attainment; nor

TABLE 28. *Significance of association of general attainment with the presence of behaviour problems in school*

Behaviour item	*Significance of level of association (χ^2) in each group*			
	Boys 5–10 yrs	*Boys 11–15 yrs*	*Girls 5–10 yrs*	*Girls 11–15 yrs*
Unco-operative in class	$P<0{\cdot}001$*	$P<0{\cdot}001$*	$P<0{\cdot}001$	$P<0{\cdot}001$
Not interested in school work	$P<0{\cdot}001$*	$P<0{\cdot}001$	$P<0{\cdot}001$	$P<0{\cdot}001$
Often tells lies	$P<0{\cdot}02$	$P<0{\cdot}001$	$P<0{\cdot}001$	$P<0{\cdot}01$
Very restless, can't sit still for a moment	$P<0{\cdot}001$	$P<0{\cdot}001$	$P<0{\cdot}01$	N.S.
Very easily frightened	$P<0{\cdot}001$	$P<0{\cdot}001$*	$P<0{\cdot}05$	$P<0{\cdot}01$
Very quiet and withdrawn	$P<0{\cdot}001$	N.S.	$P<0{\cdot}01$	$P<0{\cdot}001$
Very shy, finds it difficult to mix with other children	$P<0{\cdot}01$	$P<0{\cdot}02$	N.S.	N.S.
On one or more occasions during the school year showed fear of school—that is, tears on arrival or refusal to come into the building	$P<0{\cdot}001$	N.S.†	$P<0{\cdot}05$	N.S.†
Bites finger nails	N.S.	$P<0{\cdot}01$*	$P<0{\cdot}05$	$P<0{\cdot}001$
Sucks thumb or finger	$P<0{\cdot}01$	N.S.†	$P<0{\cdot}01$	N.S.†
Speech difficulties other than stammer	$P<0{\cdot}001$	N.S.	$P<0.001$	N.S.

* *Comparison only between 'below average' and all others.*

† *Very rare event in these groups.*

In all cases the highest frequency occurred among those with below average attainment, and the lowest frequency among the above average group. Except where otherwise stated the significance of association is based on a 3 x 2 table (i.e. 2 degrees of freedom).

was worrying any more frequent among those who had difficulty with school work.

Discussion of the child's academic achievement so far has been in terms of the individual's attainment relative to all other children of the same age and at the same type of school. It is possible, however, that this comparison does not reflect the child's actual experiences in daily school life. For instance, a child of above average attainment might nevertheless be bottom of the highest stream in the school. Similarly the 'best' pupil of the D-stream or remedial class, though a source of pride to his family, might nevertheless be below average in the wider school setting. An attempt has, therefore, been made to relate behaviour in school to achievement in the child's immediate teaching group as well as to achievement in the school as a whole.

Table 29 (page 106) shows a strong association between attainment relative to others in the same class and the underlining of behaviour problems by teachers. This is particularly marked among the boys: two out of three of the boys in the bottom quarter of the class had at least one problem underlined compared with one in three of those in the top quarter. Similarly,

TABLE 29. *Position in teaching group by number of problems of behaviour underlined by the child's teacher*

Number of items underlined by teacher	Boys						Girls					
	Position in teaching group											
	Top 25%		Middle 50%		Bottom 25%		Top 25%		Middle 50%		Bottom 25%	
	No.	%	No.	%	No.	%	No.	%	No.	%	No.	%
None	558	69	854	61	269	34	678	73	844	60	269	45
1	156	19	322	23	230	29	173	19	332	24	164	28
2	56	7	126	9	136	17	50	5	133	10	81	14
3	28	3	45	3	69	9	18	2	55	4	35	6
4 or more	14	2	52	4	76	10	9	1	31	2	44	7
Total	812	100	1399	100	780	100	928	100	1395	100	593	100

at the other end of the scale, 10 per cent of boys and 7 per cent of girls placed towards the bottom of the class had at least four items of behaviour underlined compared with 2 per cent and 1 per cent respectively of those at the top of their class ($P < 0.001$ in each case).

Relation of school behaviour to social background

Table 30 shows that among the boys there was little association between social background, as indicated by the father's occupational status, and the number of behaviour problems marked by the child's teacher. Among the girls, on the other hand, the association was highly significant. The pro-

TABLE 30. *Occupational status of father* by number of behaviour problems marked on the questionnaire by the child's teacher*

No. of items underlined by teachers	Classes 1, 2, 3		Classes 4, 5a		Class 5b		Classes 6, 7	
	Boys	Girls	Boys	Girls	Boys	Girls	Boys	Girls
None (No.)	376	447	257	287	580	621	528	408
(%)	(61%)	(70%)	(59%)	(67%)	(56%)	(61%)	(57%)	(54%)
1 (No.)	130	122	100	78	255	234	209	209
(%)	(21%)	(19%)	(23%)	(18%)	(24%)	(23%)	(23%)	(27%)
2 (No.)	67	39	46	34	107	98	80	82
(%)	(11%)	(6%)	(11%)	(8%)	(10%)	(10%)	(9%)	(11%)
3 or more (No.)	44	29	31	28	102	64	101	59
(%)	(7%)	(5%)	(7%)	(7%)	(10%)	(6%)	(11%)	(8%)
Total	617	637	434	427	1044	1017	916	758
	(100%)	(100%)	(100%)	(100%)	(100%)	(100%)	(100%)	(100%)

* *Father's occupational classification (Hall-Jones) Scale (see Table 9, page 80).*

portion of children with at least one behavioural item underlined rose steadily with diminishing occupational status from 30 per cent in the upper non-manual group to 46 per cent of those with fathers in semi-skilled or unskilled manual jobs.

Few of the individual behavioural items showed any relation to social background, and such associations as did exist varied with age and sex. 'Lack of interest in school work', for instance, was recorded for 11 per cent of boys whose fathers were in semi-skilled or unskilled manual jobs compared with only 4 per cent of those with fathers in the three highest non-manual classes, and 6 to 7 per cent of those with fathers in skilled manual or routine white-collar jobs ($P<0{\cdot}001$). This picture remained constant among boys of both primary and secondary school age. Among the girls, on the other hand, there was no variation at all with social class among the five- to ten-year-olds, of whom approximately 3 per cent showed lack of interest in each category. Among girls over the age of ten, however, the proportion of those uninterested rose steadily from 1 per cent in the professional, executive and higher supervisory group to 7 per cent among the non-skilled manual grades ($P<0{\cdot}02$).

Only three other items of behaviour showed any significant association with the father's occupation. 'Aggressiveness towards other children' was underlined for only 3 per cent of the boys aged five to ten with fathers in higher-grade non-manual jobs compared with 8 per cent of those whose fathers were semi-skilled or unskilled and 6 per cent in the other groups ($P<0{\cdot}05$). Among the girls of eleven to fifteen, the incidence of 'quiet and withdrawn' behaviour increased as the occupational status of their fathers declined: for 'professional' and 'higher non-manual' fathers it was 7 per cent, for 'lower non-manual' fathers 10 per cent; for 'skilled manual' fathers 12 per cent; and for 'semi-skilled' or 'unskilled manual' fathers 18 per cent ($P<0{\cdot}001$). In the same group of girls, nail-biting at school was also significantly associated ($P<0{\cdot}01$) with the occupational status of the father, the figures for 'professional' and 'higher non-manual', 'lower non-manual' 'skilled manual' and 'semi-skilled' or 'unskilled manual' being 2, 6, 7 and 10 per cent respectively.

Relation of school behaviour to behaviour at home

Many previous attempts to estimate the prevalence of behaviour disorders in childhood have relied solely on the information provided by teachers (e.g. Bower 1958, Cummings 1944, McFie 1934, Moore 1966, Olson 1930,

Rogers 1942, Stott 1958 and Ullman 1952). It is therefore of some importance to consider the extent to which behaviour at school may be associated with behaviour at home.

TABLE 31. *The relationship between the number of deviant behaviour items underlined by parents and the number of behaviour problems underlined by teachers*

Number of problems underlined by teachers		Number of deviant items underlined by parents							
		Boys				*Girls*			
		None	1–3	4–6	7–	None	1–3	4–6	7–
None	(No.)	740	846	108	35	817	847	135	47
	(%)	62%	55%	41%	43%	65%	61%	53%	45%
1	(No.)	259	387	62	20	283	308	68	29
	(%)	22%	25%	24%	24%	22%	22%	27%	28%
2	(No.)	115	158	43	10	107	127	24	13
	(%)	9%	10%	16%	12%	8%	9%	9%	12%
3 or more	(No.)	85	142	49	17	55	98	27	16
	(%)	7%	9%	19%	21%	4%	7%	11%	15%
Total	(No.)	1199	1533	262	82	1262	1380	254	105
Significance of association		Chi-square = 73: 9 degrees of freedom: $P<0{\cdot}001$				Chi-square = 46: 9 degrees of freedom: $P<0{\cdot}001$			

Table 31 shows that there was a significant association between the reporting of deviant behaviour* at home and of behaviour problems in school. Thus, children whose parents reported many items of deviant behaviour were about three times as likely to have multiple, i.e. three or more, problems noted by their teachers as were those reported free from deviance at home. It is, however, also obvious that the relation is not all-embracing. Nearly half of the children whose parents' assessments put them in the most deviant group were apparently free from problems at school, while more than a third of those who were without deviant behaviour at home had at least one problem recorded by their teachers.

The difference between the parents' and teachers' assessments is perhaps best illustrated if we consider the children with the highest number of behavioural items recorded in each environment. The parents' questionnaire showed that 10 per cent of children had four or more deviant items underlined: the teachers' form showed that the same proportion had three or more problems recorded. Either group of children could be taken to consist of those who were most likely to be maladjusted. However, the

* That is, behaviour reported of 10 per cent or fewer of children of the same age and sex as the child concerned. See Chapter 4, page 76.

individuals picked by each of the two methods are not the same: only about one child in five identified by one questionnaire was also identified by the other (Mitchell and Shepherd 1966).

The specific types of behaviour at school which differentiated the deviant children—i.e. those with at least four deviant items marked by their parents—from the others varied with age and sex. Table 32 shows

TABLE 32. *Behaviour items underlined significantly more often by teachers for children with four or more deviant items on the parents' questionnaire ('deviants')*

Type of behaviour underlined by teacher	*Age/sex group showing significant difference*			
	Boys		*Girls*	
	5–10 yrs	*11–15 yrs*	*5–10 yrs*	*11–15 yrs*
Easily frightened				
% of deviants	11%	5%	9%	N.S.
% of others	5%	2%	5%	
Not interested in school				
% of deviants	12%	17%	N.S.	12%
% of others	6%	5%		4%
Lying				
% of deviants	N.S.	12%	4%	4%
% of others		1%	1%	1%
Irritability				
% of deviants	N.S.	8%	6%	N.S.
% of others		3%	3%	
Thumb-sucking				
% of deviants	7%	N.S.	N.S.	N.S.
% of others	3%			
Wet/soiling				
% of deviants	5%	N.S.	N.S.	N.S.
% of others	1%			
Quiet and withdrawn				
% of deviants	17%	N.S.	N.S.	N.S.
% of others	10%			
Unco-operative in class				
% of deviants	N.S.	9%	N.S.	N.S.
% of others		2%		
Aggressive				
% of deviants	N.S.	8%	N.S.	N.S.
% of others		3%		
Worrying				
% of deviants	N.S.	8%	N.S.	N.S.
% of others		3%		
Restlessness				
% of deviants	N.S.	N.S.	11%	N.S
% of others			4%	
Stealing				
% of deviants	4%		N.S.	
% of orhers	1%			

that none of the items distinguished the deviant children from the others in all four age/sex groups. 'Lack of interest in school', 'lying' and being 'easily frightened' were the best discriminators, since they gave significantly higher figures for the deviants in three out of the four groups. The other items only distinguished deviants of one sex over a limited age range.

Chapter Seven

Changes in deviant behaviour: follow-up and findings

In the previous chapters we have presented a static picture of the distribution of the reported behavioural characteristics of the children in Buckinghamshire at one single point in time. To obtain some information about the duration as well as the intensity and frequency of deviant behaviour in this sample of children, we decided to carry out a follow-up survey in 1964, after two and a half years had elapsed.

Method

For reasons of time and finance we concentrated on reinvestigating the children who had shown most evidence of deviant behaviour in the original enquiry. In selecting this 'deviant' group of children we referred, once again, to the distribution of total deviance scores in the original sample (see table 8). Here we found that 1152 children (18 per cent) had three or more deviant items of behaviour, 687 (11 per cent) had four or more and 415 (7 per cent) had at least five. We decided that the deviant follow-up should comprise those children with four or more deviant items underlined in the questionnaires used in the original survey.* This was the highest cut-off point in terms of deviance which, even allowing for losses due to age, removal and other factors, would still provide us with an adequate number of cases for analysis.

In the original survey we only included children up to the age of fifteen. As we did not have norms of behaviour for subjects over that age and since, in any case, many of the questions we were asking would no longer have been relevant at a later age it was decided that it would be difficult in the follow-up study to judge the behavioural progress of those

* While a higher or lower cut-off point would have produced different results the decision must be determined by the nature of the research (see also Lapouse 1965, and page 159).

who had passed the school leaving age. These children were therefore necessarily excluded, thus reducing the group from 687 to 500 (260 boys and 240 girls). A second group for study was obtained by matching each 'deviant' child with another child of the same age and sex, and if possible, attending the same type and size of school, but having either no deviant behaviour item marked or, at most, only one such item.

With the help of the schools, we traced 90 per cent of the boys and 92 per cent of the girls remaining in the follow-up 'deviant' group, and 97 per cent of the boys and 92 per cent of the girls in the matched, 'deviance-free' group. Questionnaires were sent by post to the parents of 453 deviant and 474 deviance-free children.

In the original survey, the approach to parents was made, through the school but, on this occasion, the numbers involved were so much smaller that it seemed unlikely that we would find more than a few children in any one school. To single out individuals—particularly those with 'problems'—in the school setting in this way was felt to be undesirable. It was possible that the official presentation of a questionnaire to take home might cause embarrassment or anxiety to the child and suspicion on the part of the parents that the school authorities were 'picking on' their child. We therefore decided that parents should be approached directly by post, even though our pilot study (see Chapter 2) had shown that this method produced a lower response rate. The questionnaire used (see Appendix 3) contained a section on behaviour which was identical with that used in the original survey. Information sought about the child's health and family background, however, was limited to events which had taken place since the original survey, with three exceptions—age of siblings and nature and duration of permanent separation from parents—where insufficiently detailed information had been obtained originally.

Completed forms were returned by the parents of 87 per cent of the boys and 88 per cent of the girls in the deviance-free group, and by 70 per cent of the boys and 88 per cent of the girls in the deviant group. These losses meant that some of the original matched pairs in the two groups had become broken. In such cases re-matching was carried out where possible by re-pairing each unmatched deviant child with an unmatched deviance-free child of the same sex, age to within one year, and, when possible, from the same part of the county. As a result it was possible to include in the analysis the parental questionnaires for 184 pairs of boys and 193 pairs of girls.

Questionnaires identical with the teachers' forms used in the original survey were also sent to each child's class teacher and were completed for

94 per cent of the deviant and 91 per cent of the deviance-free* children respectively. Teachers' questionnaires were only included in subsequent analysis, however, if the child's parents had also completed their form.

Changes in reported behaviour

A considerable change in the distribution of deviant behaviour traits in both the deviant and deviance-free groups of children was revealed by comparison of the parent's response to the questionnaire in 1961 and in 1964 (see Table 1, page 26).

TABLE 33. *Number of deviant items underlined by parents for each child at follow-up*

No. of deviant items under-lined at follow-up	*Number of boys*		*Number of girls*	
	Deviant at original survey	*Deviance-free at original survey*	*Deviant at original survey*	*Deviance-free at original survey*
None	10	102	15	113
1	21	49	33	47
2	32	15	28	19
3	34	12	32	7
4	20	4	29	4
5	15	2	17	2
6	23	–	17	–
7	6	1	10	1
8 or more	23	–	12	–

By definition, the deviant children had all scored at least four deviant items in 1961. By 1964, 53 per cent of the boys and 56 per cent of the girls had total deviance scores which had fallen below four items; 17 per cent of the boys and 25 per cent of the girls were then entirely without such items or had only one scored. It would seem to follow, therefore, that deviant conduct was transient in a substantial proportion of children.

* It was possible to use the teachers' data to assess the extent to which the children of non-responding parents differed from those whose parents' questionnaires were completed. Out of the total of 135 non-responders, school information was available for 105 (78 per cent). This indicated that the children who could not be included in the follow-up study showed a significantly lower standard of attainment ($P < 0{\cdot}001$), a higher average amount of absence from school (thirteen sessions missed in the last full term compared with nine sessions for responders) and a slightly higher average number of behaviour problems in school (1·11 : 0·74).

A less attractive hypothesis was that the apparent improvement might merely have reflected the parents' failure to answer some items in the questionnaire, since the fewer the items answered, the greater was the probability of a low deviance score. In general, the originally deviant group were more likely to have questionnaires which contained omissions (23 per cent) than the deviance-free group (15 per cent). When, however, the presence of incomplete questionnaires among the deviant children was related to the change in the child's deviance score at follow-up, the omissions remained at a fairly constant level throughout. Thus, 24 per cent of the children with reduced scores had incomplete forms, but so had 22 per cent of those whose scores had risen.

In the originally deviance-free group, 88 per cent of the children had an initial score of zero and the remainder had only one deviant item recorded. By the time of follow-up, 18 per cent were showing at least two deviant traits and fourteen children (4 per cent) had a score of four or more items. Improvement could not be assessed in this group. By virtue of the method of selection their scores could only move in one direction, with the exception of the 12 per cent who initially had one deviant item marked. For this reason it is necessary to look separately at the changes in behaviour which occurred in each group of children.

a. Changes in the behaviour of the originally deviant group In the follow-up survey it was found that 71 per cent of boys and 74 per cent of girls had reduced total deviance scores: sixty-eight boys (37 per cent) and ninety girls (47 per cent) had reduced their scores by at least three items. At the other end of the scale there was an increased score among thirty boys (16 per cent) and twenty-one girls (11 per cent), including fourteen boys (8 per cent) and eight girls (4 per cent) who had at least three additional deviant items underlined.

TABLE 34. *Correlation between distribution of reported behaviour traits among originally 'deviant' children in 1961 and 1964*

Behaviour in 1964	*Behaviour in 1961*					
	Boys (N = 184)			*Girls* (N = 193)		
	Extreme	Moderate	Absent	Extreme	Moderate	Absent
A. THREE-POINT ITEMS						
Destructiveness						
Extreme	4	8	—	—	3	—
Moderate	7	64	18	4	33	22
Absent	—	39	39	1	32	91
	Correln. coeff. = + 0·4			Correln. coeff. = +0·4		

TABLE 34—*Continued*

Behaviour in 1964	Behaviour in 1961					
	Boys (N = 184)			*Girls* (N = 193)		
	Extreme	Moderate	Absent	Extreme	Moderate	Absent
Fear of animals						
Extreme	3	3	—	4	1	—
Moderate	5	40	13	20	42	18
Absent	1	20	91	—	36	63
	Correln. coeff. = +0·5			Correln. coeff. = +0·5		
Fear of strangers						
Extreme	2	5	—	1	3	2
Moderate	—	56	23	11	59	23
Absent	3	24	67	—	28	61
	Correln. coeff. = +0·5			Correln. coeff. = +0·4		
Fear of dark						
Extreme	17	6	2	5	11	7
Moderate	11	26	9	21	23	7
Absent	20	23	64	17	32	64
	Correln. coeff. = +0·4			Correln. coeff. = +0·3		
Lying						
Extreme	19	15	1	6	4	—
Moderate	20	104	2	6	137	7
Absent	1	9	9	3	12	14
	Correln. coeff. = +0·5			Correln. coeff. = +0·5		
Dislike of going to school						
Extreme	8	12	1	7	12	1
Moderate	11	83	22	8	65	23
Absent	4	21	19	1	31	43
	Correln. coeff. = +0·3			Correln. coeff. = +0·5		
Stealing						
Extreme	1	7	—	—	—	—
Moderate	3	47	19	—	31	19
Absent	2	23	72	—	16	119
	Correln. coeff. = +0·5			Correln. coeff. = +0·5		
Irritability						
Extreme	40	22	1	42	22	1
Moderate	35	76	4	36	76	7
Absent	—	2	1	1	4	1
	Correln. coeff. = +0·3			Correln. coeff. = +0·4		
Food fads						
Extreme	35	19	1	42	12	3
Moderate	9	28	10	20	38	14
Absent	9	16	52	8	13	41
	Correln. coeff. = +0·6			Correln. coeff. = +0·6		
Shy or afraid of other children						
Extreme	—	4	—	1	2	1
Moderate	4	36	24	4	48	23
Absent	1	24	85	3	22	87
	Correln. coeff. = +0·4			Correln. coeff. = +0·4		

TABLE 34—*Continued*

Behaviour in 1964	*Behaviour in 1961*					
	Boys (N = 184)			*Girls* (N = 193)		
	Extreme	Moderate	Absent	Extreme	Moderate	Absent
Large appetite						
Extreme	19	32	5	18	22	5
Moderate	12	69	21	16	77	22
Absent	—	7	17	—	4	28
	Correln. coeff. = +0·4			Correln. coeff. = +0·5		
Small appetite						
Extreme	17	7	—	28	4	—
Moderate	21	69	12	22	77	16
Absent	5	32	19	5	22	18
	Correln. coeff. = +0·4			Correln. coeff. = +0·5		
Worrying						
Extreme	19	15	3	17	10	1
Moderate	17	57	18	29	78	33
Absent	4	14	32	2	3	13
	Correln. coeff. = +0·5			Correln. coeff. = +0·4		
Whining, complaining						
Extreme	20	10	1	12	15	1
Moderate	26	87	10	32	92	5
Absent	3	11	11	7	11	11
	Correln. coeff. = +0.4			Correln. coeff. = +0·3		
Restlessness						
Extreme	48	21	1	48	16	1
Moderate	24	63	4	34	73	6
Absent	5	10	3	2	7	3
	Correln. coeff. = +0·4			Correln. coeff. = +0·4		
Underactivity						
Extreme	3	10	5	3	7	2
Moderate	4	63	24	6	73	34
Absent	1	21	48	1	16	48
	Correln. coeff. = +0·4			Correln. coeff. = +0·4		
Jealousy						
Extreme	20	10	2	19	10	1
Moderate	13	55	17	26	66	17
Absent	5	27	31	5	25	20
	Correln. coeff. = +0·5			Correln. coeff. = +0·4		
Wandering						
Extreme	1	9	4	1	2	1
Moderate	9	32	18	1	19	16
Absent	5	30	71	1	31	119
	Correln. coeff. = +0·3			Correln. coeff. = +0·3		
Withdrawn						
Extreme	5	7	3	2	3	—
Moderate	6	52	20	6	48	27
Absent	3	24	56	9	23	71
	Correln. coeff. = +0·4			Correln. coeff. = +0·3		

TABLE 34—*Continued*

Behaviour in 1964	*Behaviour in 1961*					
	Boys (N = 184)			*Girls* (N = 193)		
	Extreme	Moderate	Absent	Extreme	Moderate	Absent
Disobedience, resistance						
Extreme	31	23	3	33	19	1
Moderate	33	76	11	26	84	12
Absent	—	2	3	3	8	5
	Correln. coeff. = +0·3			Correln. coeff. = +0·4		
Truancy						
Extreme	—	—	—	—	—	—
Moderate	—	—	2	—	—	1
Absent	2	3	168	—	2	183
	Correln. not computed			Correln. not computed		
Twitch						
Extreme	5	1	2	—	2	1
Moderate	4	20	13	3	12	16
Absent	2	13	101	3	13	120
	Correln. coeff. = +0·6			Correln. coeff. = +0·4		
Mood changes						
Extreme	11	17	3	15	22	2
Moderate	28	72	15	21	76	14
Absent	4	16	8	3	18	12
	Correln. coeff. = +0·2			Correln. coeff. = +0·3		
Reading difficulty						
Extreme	38	12	1	18	5	—
Moderate	22	52	7	10	64	16
Absent	2	13	19	3	29	40
	Correln. coeff. = +0·6			Correln. coeff. = +0·6		

Behaviour in 1964	*Behaviour in 1961*					
	Boys			*Girls*		
	Deviant	Non-Deviant	Absent	Deviant	Non-Deviant	Absent
B. EIGHT-POINT ITEMS						
Constipation						
Deviant	11	2	2	17	6	4
Non-deviant	16	12	18	20	25	17
Absent	14	15	73	10	21	49
	Correln. coeff. = +0·4			Correln. coeff. = +0·4		
Headaches						
Deviant	17	7	5	13	8	3
Non-deviant	20	49	28	28	60	25
Absent	6	12	25	2	14	24
	Correln. coeff. = +0·6			Correln. coeff. = +0·4		

TABLE 34—*Continued*

Behaviour in 1964	*Behaviour in 1961*					
	Boys			*Girls*		
	Deviant	Non-Deviant	Absent	Deviant	Non-Deviant	Absent
Nightmares						
Deviant	12	3	7	17	11	5
Non-deviant	13	12	20	14	11	7
Absent	15	20	54	25	22	57
	Correln. coeff. = +0·3			Correln. coeff. = +0·3		
Restless in sleep						
Deviant	13	5	9	15	5	3
Non-deviant	16	19	17	15	20	19
Absent	17	21	47	14	23	56
	Correln. coeff. = +0·2			Correln. coeff. = +0·4		
Bed-wetting						
Deviant	25	2	2	12	—	5
Non-deviant	3	3	1	2	—	1
Absent	17	3	10	10	—	130
	Correln. coeff. = +0·7			Correln. coeff. = +0·6		
Stomach pains						
Deviant	24	6	8	18	6	7
Non-deviant	22	15	18	24	32	29
Absent	6	10	50	6	13	33
	Correln. coeff. = +0·5			Correln. coeff. = +0·4		
Vomiting						
Deviant	7	—	6	6	6	2
Non-deviant	6	8	11	10	9	15
Absent	9	19	87	7	16	85
	Correln. coeff. = +0·3			Correln. coeff. = +0·5		
Diarrhoea						
Deviant	10	1	8	4	4	2
Non-deviant	10	16	14	11	7	22
Absent	6	13	73	8	16	86
	Correln. coeff. = +0·4			Correln. coeff. = +0·4		
Soiling						
Deviant	8	—	1	3	—	2
Non-deviant	—	—	—	—	—	—
Absent	23	—	119	8	—	143
	Correln. coeff. = +0·4			Correln. coeff. = +0·4		
Crying						
Deviant	20	16	8	18	12	3
Non-deviant	19	35	8	24	56	16
Absent	5	33	14	7	15	15
	Correln. coeff. = +0.3			Correln. coeff. = +0·3		
Sulking						
Deviant	15	3	14	23	2	15
Non-deviant	3	1	7	3	4	7
Absent	16	2	90	18	5	82
	Correln. coeff. = +0·4			Correln. coeff. = +0·4		

TABLE 34—*Continued*

Behaviour in 1964	*Behaviour in 1961*					
	Boys			*Girls*		
	Deviant	Non-Deviant	Absent	Deviant	Non-Deviant	Absent
Tantrums						
Deviant	26	10	11	36	2	4
Non-deviant	18	19	19	18	16	13
Absent	14	18	27	18	14	40
	Correln. coeff. = +0·2			Correln. coeff. = +0·5		
Nail-biting						
Deviant	No deviant frequency			No deviant frequency		
Non-deviant		43	15		50	23
Absent		9	90		20	72
	Correln coeff. = +0·7			Correln. coeff. = +0·5		
Thumb-sucking						
Deviant	12	5	3	6	10	2
Non-deviant	—	3	1	—	17	3
Absent	6	9	117	2	7	111
	Correln. coeff. = +0·6			Correln. coeff. = +0·7		
Quarrels						
Deviant	16	5	13	21	3	13
Non-deviant	13	2	10	10	8	15
Absent	13	10	74	22	10	61
	Correln. coeff. = +0·4			Correln. coeff. = +0·3		

Table 34 (pages 114–19) illustrates the distribution of each type of behaviour in 1961 and 1964 among the originally deviant group of children and the correlation between behaviour at the two dates. It shows that there was considerable variation in the intensity of all types of behaviour over time.* The items of behaviour which showed least reported variations were, in both sexes, thumb-sucking, food fads and reading difficulties and, among the boys, nail-biting, headaches and tics. All these items appear to involve types of behaviour which persist if already present, but which do not develop readily in children of school age.

The items of behaviour showing the lowest correlations were, in both sexes, mood changes, nightmares, crying, and wandering; in girls, quarrelling with other children, fear of the dark, whining, and withdrawn behaviour; and in boys, restlessness in sleep, temper tantrums, irritability,

* In most cases the product moment correlation coefficient had a value of between +0·35 and +0·54: there was therefore a moderate amount of positive correlation between the children's behaviour in 1961 and 1964.

disobedience, dislike of going to school and vomiting. These, then, were relatively non-persistent types of behaviour which readily changed in intensity or frequency. General observation would include such forms of behaviour as possible responses to stressful situations.

So far in our discussion of the changes taking place in the behaviour of the deviant children we have dealt with the whole range of reported behaviour on each item. Comparisons have covered all the children in the group, including those who never showed the behaviour or who only showed it at moderate intensity or non-deviant frequency. Obviously, however, a special interest attaches to the persistence of 'problems' of behaviour, i.e. behaviour which occurs at extreme intensity or at a frequency deviant for children of that age and sex. Table 35 shows how many children were said to show such behaviour in 1961 and in 1964, and in how many cases the behaviour was noted on both occasions.

TABLE 35. *Persistence over time of behaviour recorded at extreme intensity or deviant frequency by originally deviant children included in the follow-up study*

1. *Behaviour shown at extreme intensity*	*No. of children showing behaviour*				*Children showing behaviour on both occasions as % of those showing it in 1961*
	(*a*) In 1961	(*b*) In 1964	(*c*) On either occasion	(*d*) On both occasions	
Destructiveness	16	15	27	4	25%
Fear of animals	33	11	37	7	21%
Fear of strangers	17	13	27	3	18%
Fear of dark	91	48	117	22	24%
Lying	55	45	75	25	45%
Dislike of going to school	39	41	65	15	38%
Stealing (all boys)	6	8	13	1	17%
Irritability	154	128	200	82	53%
Food fads	123	112	158	77	63%
Very shy of other children	13	8	20	1	1%
Large appetite	65	101	129	37	57%
Small appetite	98	66	109	45	46%
Worrying	88	65	117	36	41%
Whining	100	69	127	32	32%
Restlessness	161	135	200	96	60%
Underactivity	18	30	42	6	33%
Jealousy	88	62	111	39	44%
Wandering	18	18	34	2	11%
Withdrawn behaviour	31	20	44	7	23%
Disobedience	126	110	172	64	51%
Excessive obedience	35	21	48	8	23%
Truanting	7	3	10	Nil	Nil
Twitch or mannerism	17	11	23	5	29%
Mood changes	82	70	126	26	32%
Reading difficulty	93	74	111	56	60%
Nail-biting (daily)	77	83	113	47	61%

TABLE 35—*Continued*

2. *Behaviour shown at frequency deviant for age*[1]	*No. of children showing behaviour* (*a*) In 1961	(*b*) In 1964	(*c*) On either occasion	(*d*) On both occasions	*Children showing behaviour on both occasions as % of those showing it in 1961*
Constipation	88	42	102	28	32%
Headaches	86	53	109	30	35%
Nightmares*	96	55	122	29	30%
Restless in sleep	90	50	112	28	31%
Bed-wetting*	69	46	78	37	54%
Stomach pains	100	69	127	42	42%
Vomiting*	45	27	59	13	29%
Diarrhoea*	49	29	64	14	29%
Soiling	42	14	45	11	26%
Crying[2]	93	77	132	38	41%
Sulking	78	72	112	38	49%
Tantrums	130	89	155	62	48%
Thumb-sucking	26	38[3]	56	18	69%
Quarrels with other children	95	71	129	37	39%

[1] *As the cut-off point above which behaviour is considered deviant varies from age to age these figures should not be taken as showing the proportion of children whose behaviour is 'improving'. In the items marked * behaviour which is graded deviant may include a large range of frequencies. Thus, in bed-wetting from six years onwards practically all frequencies are deviant. A child appearing as deviant on both occasions, therefore, might actually have decreased his bed-wetting from daily frequency to once in two or three months. The degree of diminishing frequency can be seen in table 36.*

[2] *Deviance cut-off point is very closely related to age in this item.*

[3] *This apparent increase with age is due not to increased thumb-sucking but to thumb-sucking only being considered deviant from the age of eight for boys and ten for girls.*

Before discussing these findings we should perhaps reiterate that our concept of deviance is based on the occurrence of the behaviour in only 10 per cent or fewer of children of each particular age and sex. It follows, therefore, that where the prevalence of the behaviour changes as the child grows older, the definition of deviance in terms of frequency of occurrence of the behaviour will also vary. Thumb-sucking in younger children, for example, is so common that it is either not considered deviant at all or only considered deviant if it occurs very frequently; among older children, on the other hand, thumb-sucking at any frequency is rare enough to be called deviant. This means that a child who sucked his thumb every day in 1961 could have the frequency recorded as only once a month by 1964 and still figure as showing the habit at a deviant frequency on both occasions. Recorded persistence, then, does not mean that the child concerned is 'no better': it simply shows that the child is still at the same extreme of his age/sex group as he was at the time of the original survey.

Table 36 (page 122) shows that some forms of deviant behaviour were reported as far more persistent than others: at one extreme, eighteen of the twenty-six children who were sucking their thumbs at a deviant frequency

TABLE 36. *Persistence in 1964 of behaviour reported as occurring at extreme intensity or deviant frequency in 1961*

	Behaviour occurring at extreme intensity		*Behaviour occuring at deviant frequency*	
a.	*Persisting in 50% or more of the children of whom it was recorded in 1961*			
	Food fads	(63%)	Thumb-sucking	(69%)
	Daily nail-biting	(61%)	Bed-wetting	(54)%
	Restlessness	(60%)		
	Reading difficulty	(60%)		
	Large appetite	(57%)		
	Irritability	(53%)		
	Disobedience	(51%)		
b.	*Persisting in 33% or more but in less than 50% of whom it was recorded in 1961*			
	Small appetite	(46%)	Sulking	(49%)
	Lying	(45%)	Tantrums	(48%)
	Jealousy	(44%)	Stomach pains	(42%)
	Worrying	(41%)	Crying	(41%)
	Dislike of school	(38%)	Quarrels with other children	(39%)
	Underactivity	(33%)	Headaches	(35%)
			Nightmares	(33%)
c.	*Persisting in 25% or more but in less than 33% of whom it was recorded in 1961*			
	Whining	(32%)	Constipation	(32%)
	Mood changes	(32%)	Restlessness in sleep	(31%)
	Tic	(29%)	Vomiting	(29%)
	Destructiveness	(25%)	Diarrhoea	(29%)
			Soiling	(26%)
d.	*Persisting in less than 25% of whom it was recorded in 1961*			
	Fear of the dark	(24%)		
	Withdrawn behaviour	(23%)		
	Excessive obedience	(23%)		
	Fear of animals	(21%)		
	Fear of strangers	(18%)		
	Stealing	(17%)		
	Wandering	(11%)		
	Very shy of other children	(8%)		
	Truanting	(-%)		

in 1961 were still doing so in 1964; at the other extreme, all seven of the 1961 truants had reformed by 1964. Timid and withdrawn types of behaviour were among those least likely to persist. Fewer than one in four of the children who had fears, shyness, withdrawn behaviour and excessive obedience recorded in 1961 were said to exhibit such conduct at follow-up. The more delinquent types of behaviour—destructiveness, stealing, wandering and truancy—were also recorded less frequently. It would seem, therefore, that such types of deviant behaviour might reflect either a temporary phase of development or a temporary response to stress.

On the other hand, the items of behaviour which were reported as more persistent were of a different type. In the main they were either habits, e.g. thumb-sucking, nail-biting, bed-wetting, or could be seen as personality traits, e.g. restlessness, underactivity, irritability, jealousy, worrying. Reading difficulty, which was also persistent in three out of five of the children concerned, includes various types of problem—neurological, intellectual and emotional—all leading to failure to learn to read.

The physical types of 'problem'—stomach pains, headaches, constipation, vomiting, diarrhoea, soiling—appeared to fall into an intermediate position, though, even so, they were more likely to disappear than persist. Thus, only four out of every ten children who suffered from stomach pains or headaches at deviant frequency in 1961, and only three out of ten of those who vomited or had diarrhoea, were still recorded at deviant frequency in 1964.

The picture shown here is slightly different from that found when the whole range of frequency or of intensity was considered earlier (page 114). Irritability, for example, which gave a low correlation between all ranges of intensity in 1961 and 1964, showed a high degree of persistence among children who were 'very irritable'. This would appear to indicate that there was considerable alternation between moderate irritability and even-tempered behaviour in many children, but that the child described as 'very irritable' tended to go on being described in this way.

A complementary picture can be obtained by examining the development by 1964 of extreme or deviant reported items of behaviour in children of the originally deviant group who had not shown these 'problems' in 1961. In fact, the only items of behaviour of which no new cases had been reported were stealing and tics among the girls (see table 34). In general, the 'problems' most likely to develop were large appetite (17 per cent of the group), irritability, disobedience and mood changes (each 12 per cent), whining, restlessness, daily nail-biting* and crying at deviant frequency (each 9 per cent), worrying, dislike of school, fear of the dark and nightmares together with stomach pains and tantrums at deviant frequency (7 per cent). The behaviour least likely to develop included soiling, playing truant and fear of animals (1 per cent of the group in each case); acute shyness of other children, and bed-wetting at deviant frequency (2 per cent each); and destructiveness, withdrawn behaviour, fear of strangers and excessive obedience (3 per cent each).

It is also interesting to see to what extent these forms of behaviour were reported to have developed as additional items among those children whose total deviance scores has risen and to what extent they had replaced other items among those children whose total score had fallen or remained the same. In each sex there were two types of behaviour which were only

* Although possibly a 'problem', and therefore mentioned here, this would not be considered as constituting deviant behaviour at any age.

reported for the first time among children whose total deviance scores were rising and never among those whose scores were falling or constant. These were, for girls, extreme destructiveness and extreme shyness of other children; for boys, constipation and soiling, both at deviant frequency. Many other items, though found in children with falling scores, appeared to a significantly greater extent where the total score was rising. For both sexes these items were lying, worrying, whining, mood changes, tantrums and headaches ($P < 0{\cdot}001$ in all cases), disobedience, crying and quarrelling with other children; for girls only, the single item was irritability, and for boys only, underactivity and food fads ($P < 0{\cdot}01$). All these behaviour items, then, seemed more likely to develop as additional features rather than to take the place of other 'problems'.

Some other types of deviant or extreme reported behaviour seemed to develop just as readily in children whose total scores were falling. These were, in girls, dislike of going to school, underactivity, small appetite, large appetite, reading difficulty and vomiting; in boys, destructiveness, irritability, large appetite, daily nail-biting, and restlessness in sleep. Some of these items are, of course, too common to have been graded 'deviant', and their development would not affect the child's total score. Nevertheless, their appearances in children who are losing their types of deviant behaviour would indicate at least the possibility that they were replacing behaviour which had become unsuitable as the child grew older.

b. Changes in the behaviour of the originally deviance-free group At the follow-up survey in 1964 it was found that 149 (40 per cent) of the children who were originally free from deviance had developed at least one additional item of deviant behaviour. The types of such behaviour which had developed were similar to those which had appeared in the deviant group over the same period. Thus, out of the ten most frequently acquired items of deviant behaviour reported at the time of the follow-up among the originally deviant and deviance-free children, seven were common to both groups, though they did not necessarily appear in the same rank order in each case. These were nightmares, dislike of going to school, worrying, whining, stomach pains, sulking and quarrelling with other children. The type of deviant behaviour which appeared most frequently as a new item among the deviance-free group was thumb-sucking: this was recorded for 12 per cent of those with rising deviance scores, but was frequent as a new type of behaviour among the deviant group.

At the other end of the scale, none of the originally deviance-free group were said to have started to steal, play truant or soil themselves; no girls developed tics or started to tell lies and no boys began vomiting at deviant frequency. Destructiveness and extreme shyness of other children were reported in only two cases. Only four children were said to have developed fear of animals, fear of strangers, lying, tics and vomiting at deviant frequency.

Personal and environmental factors related to outcome

Since the findings presented above suggest that some items of behaviour are more likely to be transient than others, and that such forms of behaviour may be related to temporary stress it seemed logical to enquire whether certain children were more likely than others to maintain or increase their level of deviance and, if so, whether psycho-social factors were associated with outcome. As we are dealing throughout with abnormality in statistical rather than clinical terms a comparison was made between the 27 per cent of the deviant group who had not followed the general pattern of a reduction in their deviance score and the 73 per cent whose scores had diminished. We also investigated how far these two groups of children differed with respect to personal and environmental factors.* It is clearly realised that this is an artificial distinction. A child who has lost one deviant trait is not necessarily 'better' than one who has retained the same score: nevertheless, that there might be some connection is suggested by the fact that 74 per cent of children rated 'improved' in the case history study (see Chapter 9) had reduced deviance scores compared with 57 per cent of those rated 'the same' and 18 per cent of those said to be worse.

a. *Sex* There was no sex difference in the proportion of children whose total deviance scores remained the same or had risen: 29 per cent of the boys and 26 per cent of the girls fell into this category.

b. *Age* Table 37 (page 126) shows that, in most age groups, the proportion of children with decreased total deviance scores remained

* Another approach would have been to use the same type of distinction as before and compare the children who remained 'deviant' (i.e. had a total deviance score of four or more items) with those who had ceased to be so. This procedure would have identified a group of persistently deviant children. It also would have involved the combination of two separate and heterogenous groups, namely *a*) those who had remained deviant but, nevertheless, had followed the general trend by reducing their total number of deviant items of behaviour (for instance, from ten in 1961 to five in 1964); and *b*) those who remained deviant because their total deviance score was increasing. The combination of these three groups did not seem justifiable.

constant at between 70 and 80 per cent. Among the ten-year-olds, however, only 55 per cent had reduced scores. On the other hand, the group of twelve-year-olds, i.e. those who were about ten at the time of the original survey, contained the highest proportion (87 per cent) of children whose

TABLE 37. *Change in total score by age at follow-up of originally deviant children*

Age at follow up	Number and percentage of children			
	a. Whose total score had decreased		*b. Whose total score had increased or remained the same*	
	No.	%	*No.*	%
7 years	26	81	6	19
8 years	34	76	11	24
9 years	37	73	14	27
10 years	30	55	25	45
11 years	37	70	16	30
12 years	28	87	4	13
13 years	40	70	17	30
14 years	36	82	8	18
15 years	6	75	2	25
Total	274	73	103	27

scores had dropped. It would seem, then, that at the tenth year deviant items of behaviour are particularly likely to appear or to persist if already present, but that they disappear rapidly thereafter. There could be many reasons for this trend, but one general, and obvious, cause of stress at this age was the secondary selection (11-plus) examination which, in this area at this time, was first taken when the child was between nine and a half and ten and a half years old. If the first attempt was not successful, a second could be made a year later when the child was between ten and a half and eleven and a half. Walby and MacLoughlin (1963) found in Belfast that about one in five children in the qualifying year for the 11-plus examination showed 'problems' which appeared soon after they entered that year and which increased in severity up to the time of the examination. In our study, the follow-up was carried out at the time of these tests and the parents' answers may well have reflected the effects on a group of children who had already been selected as the most likely to show disorders of behaviour.

c. *Health* Only two of the health problems listed in part A of the parents' questionnaire were reported significantly more often among the children whose total score did not fall.

Among the boys (see Table 38) it appeared that those who were said

TABLE 38. *Relationship of state at follow-up to presence of hearing difficulties in boys and sick headaches in girls*

Type of health problem	*Children with 0-1 deviant traits*	*Children with 2-3 deviant traits*	*Children with 4 or more traits ('still deviant' group)* a. *Score lower than in 1961*	b. *Score more or worse than in 1961*
Boys with difficulty in hearing	3%	11%	11%	32%
Girls with sick headaches	11%	14%	26%	31%

to have 'difficulty in hearing sometimes', also maintained their high total deviance scores during the follow-up interval. In theory this association could be one of two kinds. Some children might have been suffering from a genuine loss of hearing which caused them frustration and misunderstanding at home and at school. In other cases, withdrawal and failure to respond might be attributed by parents to poor hearing so that the apparent difficulty might merely reflect the disturbance indicated by the deviance score.

Among the girls reported difficulty in hearing did not distinguish between the two groups, as it occurred only in 9 per cent of those who improved and 10 per cent of those who did not. Sick headaches, however, were associated with an increase in the deviance score and were attributed to 31 per cent of girls who had not improved compared with 14 per cent of those who had done so ($P<0{\cdot}02$).

Attendance at out-patient clinics failed to distinguish between the two groups, in both of which the majority of such attendances had been for physical complaints. Behaviour problems and 'nervousness' had, however, involved out-patient treatment for eight of the ninety-eight children who were regarded as the same or 'worse' (8 per cent) compared with five out of the 278 (2 per cent) of those who were 'better'. Similarly, five out of the seven children treated by their family doctors for behaviour problems came from the group who had failed to improve.

d. *School background* The children whose total deviance scores were not recorded as having improved did not seem to differ from the others in respect of academic attainment. They did, however, have a slightly poorer attendance record; 70 per cent had lost five or more half-day sessions during the previous term, compared with 55 per cent of the rest ($P<0{\cdot}02$). Most of the differences seemed to be due to a higher incidence of short absences from school in those whose behaviour score had not decreased; absence of more than three weeks during the term was found equally in both groups.

Teachers tended to underline slightly fewer behaviour items as applying to the group whose total score on the parents' questionnaire had dropped (average 0·9) than to the others (average 1·2). The most frequently underlined items among those who had failed to improve were: 'very quiet and withdrawn' (18 per cent); 'worries more than other children' (12 per cent); 'finds it difficult to mix with other children' (11 per cent); 'restless, can't sit still for a moment' (11 per cent); 'very easily frightened' (8 per cent) 'often tell lies' (7 per cent); 'very moody' (6 per cent); and, 'not interested in school work' (6 per cent). Three types of item, all quite uncommon, were closely related to failure to improve, inasmuch as more than the reported cases fell in the group of children who were regarded as unchanged or worse. These were: 'cries more than other children' (3/5 children); 'has noticeable twitch of face or body' (4/4 children); and 'fear of school or school refusal' (3/3 children). At the other end of the scale, aggressiveness towards other children, nail-biting, and unco-operative conduct in class were relatively common among those who improved and rare among those who did not.

e. Family background Parents' occupations appeared to bear little relationship to whether or not a child's total deviance score declined. Thus, 73 per cent of boys whose fathers were in manual occupations had reduced scores; in the non-manual group the proportion was 69 per cent. Among the girls, 70 per cent of the manual group had lower scores compared with 80 per cent of the non-manual.

Similarly, there appeared to be no consistent relation between changes in the mother's working day and changes in the children's scores (Table 39). The proportion of girls whose scores had decreased remained constant, regardless of changes in the mother's work pattern. Among the boys, however, only 50 per cent of those whose mothers were working longer hours had reduced scores compared with 74 per cent of the sons of those working the same or fewer hours ($P < 0{\cdot}02$).

Neither family position nor number of siblings showed any relation to changes in total score. Only twenty-six boys and forty-four girls had had a new sibling born into the family since the original survey, and of these children, approximately 70 per cent of each sex had reduced scores.

Similarly, there was no evidence to show that bereavement had occurred to a greater extent among the children whose scores remained

TABLE 39. *Change in total deviance score by change in mother's hours of employment*

Change in mother's working hours	*Child's score decreased at follow-up*				*Child's score the same or increased*			
	Boys		*Girls*		*Boys*		*Girls*	
	No.	%	*No.*	%	*No.*	%	*No.*	%
Same as before*	90	73	101	73	33	27	37	27
Working more than before	16	50	18	72	16	50	7	28
Working less than before†	10	83	11	73	2	17	4	27
No mother or insufficient data	15	88	13	87	2	12	2	12
Total children	131		143		53		50	

* *Including those not working at all on either occasion.*
† *Including those who had stopped working.*

unchanged or had increased; about one in five of the girls in each group, and about one in four of the boys, had suffered the death of a relative or close friend during the follow-up period. Most of these deaths had taken place among grandparents.

Illness had occurred among other members of the household in 38 per cent of the children whose scores remained the same or increased, compared with 33 per cent of those whose scores had dropped. There was no difference in the proportion of fathers who had been ill: this remained constant at 6 per cent in each group and each sex. The mothers of boys whose scores had not decreased were slightly more likely to have been admitted to hospital (13 per cent) than were those of the other boys (9 per cent); there was no difference among the girls (13 per cent of mothers in each group). Only nine fathers were reported to have been sick at home but, of these, seven belonged to children who had failed to improve. Psychiatric illness, which had been treated either at home or in hospital, was recorded as affecting three fathers and four mothers and, in all but one case, the children had a reduced deviance score at the time of the follow-up.

It appears, then, that investigation of environmental changes during the follow-up period failed to discriminate between children whose scores had and had not fallen. It was not possible, however, to measure more subjective changes by means of the questionnaire investigation. This was one of the objects of the more detailed individual study which is described in Chapters 8 and 9.

Chapter Eight

Psychiatric treatment 1: referral to child guidance clinics

The results of the random sample survey made it clear that there were many children in the county whose reported behaviour patterns suggested a considerable degree of disturbance. It was equally obvious that virtually none of these children had been referred for psychiatric help.* This is not a novel observation. As early as 1925, Haggerty pointed out: 'The stream of behaviour children which day by day flows through a Child Guidance Clinic suggests to any careful observer two things: first, that in our school population there are a far larger number of behaviour children than most of us would have believed and, second, that the variety of behaviour symptoms ranges through many forms.'

Preston and Shepler (1930) took full psychiatric and social histories for forty-five children aged seven and a half to eight and a half years, comprising one whole class in an above-average city public school in America; none of these children had been referred for psychiatric treatment, attended Juvenile Court or been noted by their teachers as showing any outstanding problems of behaviour. The case histories were then sent, in batches of three, to fifteen separate psychiatric clinics with a request for an opinion whether the children required psychiatric help. In the view of the clinic doctors seventeen (38 per cent) of these forty-five children should have been referred for treatment.

A generation later the situation appears to be essentially unchanged. Thus a family doctor with a strong interest in psychiatric problems (Ryle 1963) has reported, 'in my own practice, for each child referred to child guidance (and I refer 8 per cent, ten times the national average) there are five, equally disturbed, not referred'. It is reasonable to enquire why so few children with disturbances of behaviour are referred to clinics, and why comparable cases are so referred. Our sample survey, by providing a comprehensive picture of children's behaviour, gave us an

* Out of a total sample of 6303 children, nine were reported as receiving or having received psychiatric treatment.

opportunity of considering these important questions, for we were able to contrast children who had been referred to child guidance clinics with a suitable control group drawn from the main sample. These children were matched with the clinic attenders for age, sex and deviant behaviour but were drawn from those who had never been referred for psychiatric treatment.

SELECTION OF CHILDREN ATTENDING CLINICS

To compare the factors which led some children to attend clinics while others with similar behaviour problems were not referred, it was decided to interview the parent of each consecutive new patient* arriving at any of the three clinics then operating in the county. These interviews were arranged to take place on the child's first visit to the clinic, or as soon as possible thereafter. At this time it could be reasonably assumed that the parents would still retain their original attitudes both towards their children's problems and towards attendance at a child guidance clinic, but they would also have established contact with the clinic staff.

Two other possibilities were considered and rejected. If we had taken a sample of children who were already receiving treatment then both the child's behaviour and the parents' reaction to it might have been altered by contact with the clinic. Again, if the children had been taken from those who were newly referred, we could have obtained a clearer picture of the relevant factors determining the referral but a long time usually elapsed between referral and treatment; it was felt that asking for information while withholding help during this time would have been undesirable on ethical grounds.

Because we intended to compare the clinic children with those from the main survey, we excluded from our inquiry all those cases for whom we could find no counterparts in the sample: those who were under or over statutory school age and those who were unable to attend an ordinary school because of physical or mental handicaps. Since we were interested in the factors affecting voluntary attendance at clinics we also decided to omit children referred by juvenile courts and those already in residential care. Other exclusions were due to refusals, administrative difficulties, etc. At two of the clinics, losses amounted to two children whose mothers refused to be interviewed for the purposes of our research; one child who was not available because he left the area immediately

* These were the children who had not previously attended any other child guidance clinic themselves and who had no other member of their family already attending the same clinic.

after his first visit to the clinic; and three children who were treated by home visits by the clinic staff. In the third clinic, access was limited to cases in which members of the clinic staff felt that a research interview would not interfere with their own relations with the family. This eliminated seventeen children whom, judging from clinic case-notes, it would have been possible to match from the main sample: fourteen children were included in our study. A fourth clinic was opened during the time when we were collecting cases but, because of administrative difficulties, it was only possible to get in touch with the parent of one out of the first seven matchable children attending.

TABLE 40. *Reasons for exclusion of children attending child guidance clinics for the first time during the period of the survey**

Reason	*Number of children*	
	Boys	*Girls*
Aged less than 5 years	8	4
Aged more than 15 years	1	3
Problem due to epilepsy, psychosis or brain damage	4	–
Problems unmatched	7	8
Child referred through court or probation officer	5	–
Child in residential care (children's home, school, etc.)	4	2
Child already being treated elsewhere	1	–
Siblings already being treated by the clinic	1	2
Total in excluded categories	31	19

* *This only included children accepted for treatment. In addition, some children were seen for psychometric testing or a psychiatric opinion at the request of local paediatricians, and two children were referred by their family doctors but were not regarded by the psychiatrist as showing any psychiatric abnormality.*

The fifty cases finally included in the study comprised about two-thirds of those who would have been eligible. A study of referral notes and clinic case histories did not suggest that those included differed in any significant respect from the matchable cases who were omitted. Our cases did not, however, include the most seriously disturbed children who had been referred to clinics during the period covered by the study since thirty (27 per cent) of the total 112 new cases were excluded as unmatchable. This is a generous estimate as it includes children in care of the local authority who, in terms of symptoms, may not have been worse than the matchable children. The cases studied were probably typical of about three out of four children of school age attending child guidance clinics. Even if the matchable children who were omitted had been more disturbed, those who were included would still have been representative of at least half of all school-age patients.

INTERVIEWING THE PARENTS OF CLINIC ATTENDERS

The parents of each of the children included in the study were asked initially to tell their own story of the 'problem' which had brought them to the clinic. Questions at this stage were limited to clarification of terminology ('What exactly happens when she has a "dizzy turn"?'), frequency ('How often does that happen?'), duration ('How long has he been doing that?'), or possible causation ('When does she usually get the pain?'), etc. Details were also obtained about the child's background including age, occupation and mental and physical health of the parents, number and age of siblings, details of the child's health and life-experiences, e.g. separation, present housing situation, and the parent's views on the child's adjustment and progress at school. The parent also completed one of the questionnaires used in the main sample inquiry.

MATCHING OF CLINIC CASES

A punched card was prepared for each clinic child showing age, sex and each item of behaviour which had been underlined on our questionnaire by his parent. A special note was made on each card of the problems which the parents regarded as most important in leading to the child's referral to the clinic. We then sorted all the sample survey cards for children of appropriate age and sex and extracted those with the same main problem or problems as the clinic child. In some cases the match was obvious, but where there were several possibilities, we referred to the original questionnaires and checked for closeness of age, school attainment and social background as well as behaviour; in every instance, however, behaviour was the main determinant. In some cases where the problem was not specifically covered by the questionnaire (for example, masturbation or nail-picking), we matched by using information given under the general heading of 'Any other worries about the child's behaviour or habits'. In other cases, where the referral problems were connected with behaviour at school, we used the teachers' questionnaires.

INTERVIEWS WITH PARENTS OF CHILDREN NOT ATTENDING CLINICS

Once a child had been selected as a suitable match for a clinic patient, a letter was written to the child's parents explaining the purpose of the more detailed, personal investigation and suggesting a suitable time for visiting them at home. Two parents, both of girls who had started work, said they did not wish to be interviewed and a further nine were not at home when visited. In these cases we used the next best match.

All the interviews took place at home, usually with the mother during school hours while the children were out, but also in the evening or on Saturday mornings if the mother was working or if the father also wanted to be present. We explained to the parents that we were interested in the type of problems which people met in bringing up their children and the extent to which parents received help in dealing with such problems. In many cases this initial explanation, without further prompting, evoked a long story dealing with family relations as well as the child's behaviour. This account provided the most useful basis for further, more detailed, enquiries but, where the mother was more reticent or found it difficult to express herself, she was taken step-by-step through the interview schedule and questioned about the answers she had given on her original questionnaire.

The case histories set out in Appendix 2 (page 175) illustrate the type of information obtained and the quality of matching.

Comparison of the child guidance children and their matched controls

I. SEVERITY OF DISTURBANCE

It quickly became apparent that, though all clinic children might be considered 'disturbed', since otherwise they would not have been referred, there was nevertheless a considerable variation in the severity of their disturbance. To obtain some form of clinical rating of the degree of disturbance a case history, based on the parent's information, was compiled for each child and five raters* then each made an independent assessment of each case history. None of the raters was connected with the survey and none treated children from the area studied. Only the typewritten case history of each child, together with information about his or her age and sex, was provided. Neither the purpose of the rating nor the source of the information was disclosed, and all references to treatment were omitted. Each profile was numbered from 1 to 100 by the use of random

* These were two consultant psychiatrists, two psychiatric senior registrars and one psychologist/psychotherapist. All had experience in child psychiatry, and one consultant and both senior registrars were currently working in child guidance clinics.

number tables and the set of case histories was presented to each rater in numerical order so that no clues would be provided about the matching procedure.

The raters were asked to use a five-point scale as follows: very severely disturbed (score = 5); severely disturbed (score = 4); moderately disturbed (score = 3); mildly disturbed (score = 2); very mildly disturbed (score = 1).

TABLE 41. *Correlation between raters on degree of disturbance shown by 100 children*

Rater	A	B	C	D	E
A	—	+·34[3]	·25[1]	+·11	+·38[3]
B	+·34[3]	—	·65[3]	+·37[3]	+·41[3]
C[4]	+·25[1]	+·65[3]	—	+·21[1]	+·31[2]
D[4]	+·11	+·37[3]	+·21[1]	—	+·43[3]
E[4]	+·38[3]	+·41[3]	+·31[2]	+·43[3]	—

1 *Significantly different from zero at P<0·05.*
2 *Significantly different from zero at P<0·001.*
3 *Significantly different from zero at P<0·001.*
4 *Rater currently on the staff of a child guidance clinic.*

As table 41 shows, there was only moderate agreement between the raters. Considered in closer detail, ratings for a particular child varied from 'very mild' to 'moderate' in twenty-four cases and from 'very mild' to 'severe' in two cases. There was complete agreement between all five raters in only three cases; agreement by at least four out of five in twenty cases, and agreement by at least three raters in fifty-nine cases. We had deliberately not laid down any guide lines for raters in terms of percentages or other definitions since we wanted them to proceed as they would on receiving a report on a child referred to their clinic, using their own criteria of disturbance. As a result one of the main reasons for variation appeared to lie in differences in the frames of reference employed. For instance, one rather felt that 'very severely disturbed' should be applied to 'psychotic or frankly psychopathic' children, whereas another would use it for those 'likely to develop serious mental illness in adult life'. Others found it difficult to define their criteria at all without resource to descriptions of particular types of behaviour which to them would be indicative of serious disturbance. In fact, the lack of agreement shown by the raters indicates only too clearly the difficulty of defining the characteristics of a 'disturbed' child in any generally acceptable way.

TABLE 42. *Average rating score* of children referred to clinics and matched non-referred children*

Average rating score	*Clinic attenders*	*Non-clinic group*
1 ('very mild')	1	1
2 ('mild')	12	23
3 ('moderate')	29	22
4 ('severe')	8	4
	50	50

* *Obtained by giving each a score as shown in brackets on page 135, and then computing the average score for each child.*

It can be seen from table 42 that while the children attending clinics tended to be given a more severe average rating than their controls, this difference was not statistically significant ($\chi^2 = 5{\cdot}00$: d.f. $=2$: $0{\cdot}10 > P > 0{\cdot}05$). A comparison of the two children of each matched pair showed that in twenty-seven pairs both children had the same rating and that in a further eleven pairs there was a difference of less than five points in the *total* rating score, i.e. the combined score given to him by all five raters. This means that in three-quarters of the matched pairs both children were given the same rating by at least one rater. In the remaining twelve pairs there was general agreement that the clinic child was the more disturbed in eleven cases when he or she had an average rating of three (moderate) or four (severe) compared with the non-clinic child's rating of two (mild) in all eleven instances. Yet though it might be argued, then, that mildness of disturbance was the main reason for non-referral (Wolff 1967) in one in five of the matched cases even this is by no means certain, since table 42 shows that one in four of the clinic referrals also had an average rating of two.

A similar picture emerged when the two groups were compared in respect of statistical deviance. Of the fifty children in each group, forty of the clinic attenders and thirty-seven of the non-clinic children had four or more deviant items scored on the parents' questionnaire. In each group, all but three of the children with a deviance score of less than four were given average ratings indicative of only mild disturbance.

It appeared, then, that for the majority of children neither the clinical nor the statistical methods of assessing abnormality indicated that degree of disturbance was the main factor leading to referral for psychiatric treatment.

2. ENVIRONMENTAL FACTORS

a. Ease of access to clinics Before the parents were interviewed it was possible to set up several hypotheses about the environmental factors which might explain why one child reached a clinic while another did not. The most obvious of these in a large, and to a great extent rural area, sparsely provided with clinics, was that some children were geographically separated from a convenient clinic. There was no evidence to support this suggestion: 42 per cent of those attending a clinic lived in one of the towns where a clinic was held and so did 42 per cent of non-clinic children. At the other end of the scale five clinic children (10 per cent) and two non-clinic children (4 per cent) had either a long or a difficult journey to the nearest clinic.

Even with an apparently easy journey, however, a mother might have been unable to bring a child to a clinic because of other demands on her time: for example, other young children in the family or inability or unwillingness to take time off from work. The presence of young children in the household did not appear to deter families from attending clinics: among the girls, eight in each group had siblings of pre-school age, and among the twenty-nine pairs of boys twelve of the clinic attenders fell into this category compared with only seven non-clinic boys.

Among the girls there was no difference in the number of mothers employed in each group (40 per cent), but among the boys there was a slightly higher proportion of working mothers among those whose sons did not attend a clinic: fifteen compared with nine of the clinic boys. This difference is not significant and the interviews provided no evidence of work being given priority over the children's interests. Indeed, in two cases, mothers of non-clinic boys took time off work, with resultant loss of pay, to be interviewed for the survey.

b Socio-economic factors The socio-economic status of the two groups of children, as indicated by the occupational class of the father, differed significantly ($\chi^2 = 4{\cdot}76$; d.f. $= 1$: $P < 0{\cdot}05$): the proportion of fathers in non-manual occupations was twice as great among the clinic children (40 per cent) as among the non-clinic children (20 per cent). The difference was particularly marked in the 'higher' strata of each occupational group. Sixteen of the clinic children had fathers in managerial or higher supervisory types of job (Hall-Jones classes 2 and 3) compared with five of those not attending clinics; twenty-five non-clinic children had fathers in skilled manual jobs compared with sixteen of those attending clinics. The proportion whose fathers were in routine white-collar or semi-skilled or un-skilled jobs was much the same in each group. It is tempting to suggest that these findings may show a greater knowledge and use of psychiatric services by the more educated parent, but further investigation rendered this explanation unlikely. Thus of the ten boys attending clinics whose fathers were in occupational classes 2 or 3 (there were none in class 1), the parents had asked for child guidance referral in only one case.* In two cases, the child was first taken to a paediatrician and in two cases, through the family doctor, to an adult psychiatric out-patient clinic. In four cases, the suggestion of child guidance came first from the head teacher at the child's school† and, in the last case, from the family doctor.

The differences in social class are more likely to reflect the methods by which the control group was selected. It was taken from the main sample of pupils at local authority schools, and by excluding private school pupils, there has certainly been some exclusion of children in social classes I and II.

c. *Familial factors* There was no evidence to support hypotheses relating referral to the age of the parents on grounds of *a* lessened tolerance with increasing age; *b* increased tolerance with increasing experience; or *c* greater resistance to psychiatric help on the part of older parents. The average age of mothers at the child's birth was 28·0 years for clinic boys and 27·5 years for non-clinic boys; 24·5 years for clinic girls and 25·9 years for non-clinic girls. It might be argued that the mother's age at the time of the child's birth is less important in this context than her age at the time of the survey. Here again, however, there was little difference; 27 per cent of the mothers of clinic children and 33 per cent of those of the non-clinic group were over forty years of age.

The position in the family was similar for both groups of children except that the non-clinic group contained a slightly higher proportion of those who were the youngest living children in their family and a slightly lower proportion of only children; in each group twenty-two children were the surviving eldest in the family and thirteen clinic and twelve non-clinic children were middle children.

Similarly, the total size of the family showed no consistent relation to whether or not the child attended a clinic. Among the boys five clinic

* This was the case of a five-year-old boy whose parents were convinced, mistakenly, that he had an emotional block to learning and was not 'backward' as suggested by his school.

† In two cases this involved threats of exclusion from school unless advice was sought by the parents.

children and two non-clinic children had four or more siblings; among the girls, all those attending clinics had fewer than four siblings whereas five of the non-clinic group had four or more.

d. Separation experiences Clinic children had suffered considerably more family disruption through death or desertion than had their non-clinic counterparts. Among clinic children, ten had lost at least one parent permanently compared with three in the non-clinic group. This was particularly true of paternal loss among the boys since six clinic boys had lost their fathers by desertion, divorce, etc., whereas none of the non-clinic group had done so (by Fisher's exact 2-tailed method, $P = 0{\cdot}0186$). The clinic children also were slightly more likely to have lost an older sibling (seven cases) than the non-clinic (three cases). These numbers are, however, very small.

Separation amounting to more than two months spent away from home had been experienced by seven clinic children and three non-clinic children. This is probably to some extent a reflection of the family disruption already discussed, as about half the children concerned had also lost a parent.

Similar proportions of the two groups of boys had experienced at least one admission to hospital but thirteen of the clinic girls had been admitted to hospital, compared with eight of the non-clinic girls, and this trend was consistent for all durations of stay.

e. Inter-personal factors. In terms of the objectively ascertainable background factors, therefore, the differences between clinic attenders and non-attenders were small. The clinic attenders were more likely to have had fathers in non-manual types of occupation, and were more likely to have lost a parent and to have had an older sibling who died, in most cases at birth or shortly afterwards. If they were girls, they were more likely to have been hospital in-patients; if boys, to have lost their fathers, to have experienced a long separation from home and to have had mothers who were not employed at the time of attending clinic.

It appeared likely, then, that if any marked differences did exist between the families of clinic and non-clinic children, they must lie among less tangible factors such as family relations and parent's attitudes. This view was reinforced when we looked at the parents', usually the mothers', reactions to the children's behaviour, and the action taken to deal with it.

Here, as can be seen in table 43 the most obvious difference lay in the number of mothers of non-clinic children who, while noticing that their children had problems, felt that these were unavoidable (for both sexes

TABLE 43. *Parental attitudes to child's behaviour*

Parental attitudes	*Number of boys* Clinic N = 29	*Number of boys* Non-clinic N = 29	*Number of girls* Clinic N = 21	*Number of girls* Non-clinic N = 21
Exasperation, irritation, shame (including general rejection where the child was resented in all ways)	13	14	10	4
Worry about child's welfare (including poor school progress) or unhappiness[2]	10	5	10	3
Helpless, puzzled, unable to cope (or parental disagreement as to method)[1]	5	2	7	1
Fear of delinquency or Court proceedings (for absence from school, etc.)	3	1	2	1
Problem identified but considered unavoidable because of environmental or developmental factors[2]	—	5	1	10
Problems regarded as physical	—	3	—	4
Problems regarded as educational	—	1	—	—
No problem admitted to exist in child's behaviour	2[3]	2	1[3]	2

1 *For both sexes combined, difference between clinic and non-clinic groups significant at $P<0{\cdot}05$.*

2 *For both sexes combined, difference between clinic and non-clinic groups significant at $P<0{\cdot}001$.*

3 *Attended because of pressure from the child's school.*

combined, $\chi^2 = 12{\cdot}6$: d.f. = 1: $P<0{\cdot}001$). 'She's just going through a phase, I suppose', was the dominant theme among these mothers—often accompanied by 'but I wish she'd get over it'. On the whole, however, they felt that the only thing to do was to 'let it wash over us'. Another mother felt that it was the result of her daughter's horoscope that she should be 'difficult'. This general feeling that problems must be accepted as a necessary part of child-rearing was particularly obvious among the mothers of girls not attending clinics, where it was shown by just under half. Only one mother of a clinic child felt this way and she had arrived at the clinic as the result of an accident.*

Mothers of children who were referred to clinics were much more likely to feel worried about their children's problems. In some cases this worry was associated with the child's present unhappiness, e.g. 'I'm afraid she might do something silly.' In others, the worry went with future

* This girl had been vomiting every school morning for years and her mother felt the vomiting must just be accepted as a fact of life after so long. She was referred to the child guidance clinic by a paediatrician who heard of her vomiting when she was admitted to hospital as a result of accidental poisoning through an error in prescription.

prospects, e.g. 'What's going to become of him if he goes on like this?' Clinic mothers also felt more puzzled and helpless about coping with their children's problems: 'You lie awake wondering what you've done wrong'; 'I'm at my wits' ends'; 'His Dad says he needs a good thrashing, but I don't know if that's the best way'.

Mothers of clinic-attending girls also showed a greater tendency to feel irritated with their daughters' behaviour, e.g. 'You can't get your work done with a child stamping her feet and shouting at you all the time. I sometimes think they'll have to shut her up—or me!' Such differences were not significant, however, and did not apply at all in the case of boys. Perhaps as a result of their different attitudes, parents of children attending clinics were also more likely to have sought advice about their children's behaviour. For example, 62 per cent had discussed their problems with the child's teacher (or head teacher) compared with only 26 per cent of the non-clinic group ($\chi^2 = 6{\cdot}00$: d.f. $= 1$: $P < 0{\cdot}02$). Probably as a result of these discussions 26 per cent of the clinic attenders had also consulted the school doctor, compared with 4 per cent of the non-clinic children ($\chi^2 = 7{\cdot}80$: d.f. $= 1$: $P < 0{\cdot}01$). A large proportion of parents in both groups had consulted their family doctor: 70 per cent of the clinic group, 60 per cent of the others.

The parents of children attending clinics also reported more frequently that they used punishment in dealing with their children's problems; this had been used by the parents of 44 per cent of clinic attenders and only 18 per cent of those of the non-clinic group ($\chi^2 = 6{\cdot}72$: d.f. $= 1$: $P < 0{\cdot}01$). The mothers of six other clinic boys adopted the method of deliberately ignoring the child's behaviour, but this did not occur at all among either the girls attending clinics or the non-clinic group.

The non-clinic mothers were much more likely to feel that they supplied reassurance, encouragement and support for their children ($\chi^2 = 9{\cdot}94$: d.f. $= 1$: $P < 0{\cdot}01$). Several such mothers attributed the child's problems to his or her ordinal position in the family and tried to compensate for this, e.g. 'I think he does it to make himself important. He feels a bit pushed out, being in the middle, so I try to take a special interest in what he is doing'; 'It's hard on her (as the eldest of five children), with the little boys making a noise when she wants to do her homework and that, so I give her some extras and a bit of fussing when they're in bed'.

Such reports, of course, only indicated the mother's own perception of the way in which she dealt with her child. Her views do not necessarily coincide with actual events, as has been shown by Crandall and Preston (1955) and Gordon (1957). There did, however, appear to be fairly consistent patterns in the self-perceptions of the two groups. The non-clinic mothers tended to a greater extent to be able to accept their children's behaviour and to feel capable of dealing with it themselves; the clinic group were more likely to worry about the child's problems and to seek advice.

In looking at their own health, mothers of clinic attenders were more likely to see themselves as 'suffering from nerves' than were non-clinic mothers. In particular, they were more likely to complain that they often felt worried (fourteen clinic mothers; six of the non-clinic): they were easily upset by stressful situations to which they responded by fainting, by developing pains or diarrhoea, or by vomiting; they felt mildly depressed, tired and unappreciated and found it difficult to cope with their daily round of house, husband and children.

Irritability and quickness of temper were mentioned by about one in four of mothers of both clinic and non-clinic children. Similarly, there was no difference in the prevalence of more serious symptoms. In each group, eight mothers had suffered from psychiatric illness to a degree which had limited their social or business life—fear of leaving the house, or meeting people, going into shops—or which had necessitated treatment by their family doctor or a psychiatrist, e.g. depression associated with childbirth. In all these cases, the illness had either occurred in the recent past or still existed at the time of interview.

Fathers of the children attending clinics, on the other hand, were less likely to be regarded as suffering from 'nerves' (27 per cent) than those of non-clinic children (45 per cent). In most cases, of course, this impression is entirely based on the wife's view. Further, the circumstances if the interviews differed. The clinic-attending mothers knew that their child was felt to need psychiatric help and may, therefore, have felt chary about discussing their husband's failings lest this resulted in the father being 'blamed' for the child's condition. They did not, however, appear to feel any such scruples about discussing their own irritability or anxieties.

When the 'nerves' of both parents were considered in combination, there was little difference between the parents of the two groups of girls. Among the boys, however, there was a tendency for the non-clinic mothers to attribute 'nerves' to their husbands but not to themselves (six non-clinic cases, no clinic-attenders); conversely, more clinic mothers saw themselves as having 'nerves' while their husbands did not (twelve clinic mothers, none of the others).

These views of the situation are, of course, entirely subjective. Thus the mother who described herself as placid but married to a 'difficult' or excessively irritable man was only presenting her view of the situation;

the husband might equally well see himself as a patient and tolerant man married to an infuriatingly ineffectual wife. It is interesting to note, however, that the mother's view of the family situation as reported here supports our findings in relation to the mother's reactions to the child's behaviour problems. In both fields, the non-clinic mothers appeared to see themselves as coping more positively with the difficulties of life, including their husbands' 'nerves', than did mothers of children who attended clinics.

Chapter Nine

Psychiatric treatment 2: a controlled follow-up study of children attending child guidance clinics

In the main sample follow-up study (see Chapter 7) it was shown that deviations from 'normal' behaviour tended to be temporary and to remit over time. This finding raises several important questions for the planning of child guidance services. How far can one expect children's behaviour disorders to resolve themselves spontaneously? To what extent is treatment necessary? Are certain types of background or certain types of problems more likely to result in spontaneous remission than others? And can a reduction in the number of deviant items reported be used as an index of improvement in mental health?

In an attempt to suggest at least provisional answers to these questions we decided to interview the parents of the clinic children and their matched controls once again after an interval of about two years.

Methods

APPROACHING THE PARENTS

We were able to interview forty-four clinic parents and forty-three non-clinic parents out of a possible fifty in each case. The parents of four clinic children did not wish to be interviewed again and the other two, who were still receiving treatment, were dropped at the request of the doctor concerned. Among the seven sets of non-clinic parents who could not be interviewed again, one family had emigrated and one had moved to a distant part of the country. The other five children were traced but one mother did not wish to be interviewed as her boy had been sent to an approved school. The other four mothers were not to be found at home; three were known to be working full time and the fourth was probably hiding as her husband had just been sent to prison.

The interview schedule was designed to give a picture of changes which had occurred in the child's behaviour and in the family environment. This was supplemented by completion, during the interview, of the same questionnaire which was used in the main follow-up study. This made it possible to carry out a comprehensive analysis of any changes in behaviour which had taken place.

ASSESSMENT OF THE CHILD'S STATE

As before (see page 134), a report was prepared embodying the parent's description of the child's behaviour. These reports, together with the original case history in each case, were presented to three of the raters (two of the child psychiatrists and the psychologist) who had assessed the original state of the children, since the other two were unavailable. In each case the assessor was also provided with the assessment that he had given on the child's original state. The rating of change was given on a five-point scale as follows: 'definitely improved' (+ 2); 'slightly improved' (+ 1); 'the same' (0); 'slightly worse' (— 1); 'definitely worse (— 2). All references to the treatment received by the child were again omitted, and the raters had no means of knowing which children had attended psychiatric clinics. As can be seen in table 44, the agreement between the three raters on the relative improvement or deterioration was much closer than it had been on the original ratings (see page 135).

TABLE 44. *Correlation between raters on degree of improvement/deterioration shown by the eighty-seven children included in the follow-up*

Rater	B	D	E
B	—	+·83	+·60
D	+·83	—	+·60
E	+·60	+·60	—

In each case the correlation coefficient was significantly different from zero at the 0·1 per cent level of probability.

Only fragmentary information was available about the remaining thirteen children whose parents had not been interviewed for a second time. Of those who had originally attended clinics, one girl was being treated for a recurrence of school phobia at a clinic in another county; two girls were receiving psychotherapy and, according to their therapist, improving; one boy, a ticqueur, was said by his mother in a letter to be 'doing well' in an office; another ex-high school girl had had a rather varied career, according to her brother, and was working in a shop; nothing was known of the sixth child as he had moved out of the county. Of the non-clinic children, one boy had been sent to an approved school; one was still showing seven 'deviant' items on the parents' questionnaire and was said by his school to worry more than usual for boys of his age; one boy was said by his teacher to have 'too much money and too little discipline at home'; another appeared quite unexceptional to his teachers; and nothing was known of the other two boys as they had left the county and, in one case, the country as well. The only non-clinic girl whose mother was not interviewed appeared to be doing quite well at school, despite family upheaval due to her father's conviction and imprisonment.

ASSESSMENT OF CLINICAL STATE AT FOLLOW-UP

In both groups the ratings at follow-up indicated an improvement in just over three-fifths of the children and, as table 45 shows, there were no marked differences between the changes in each group.

TABLE 45. *State at follow-up of children in original clinic-attending and non-clinic groups*

Average improvement/deterioration rating at follow-up	*Clinic-attending children*		*Matched children*	
	No.	%	*No.*	%
Improved	29	65	26*	61
Unchanged	8	18	13*	30
Worse	7	16	4	9

* *Including one child in each category who had been referred to a child-guidance clinic during the follow-up interval and had received treatment.*

$\chi^2 = 2{\cdot}81$: *d.f.* = 2: *not significant.*

A further analysis showed there to be no consistent relationship between the child's state at follow-up and the number of times on which he or she had attended a clinic.★ Thus, of the twenty-one children who had attended up to five times, seventeen (85 per cent) had improved; of the twelve with six to fifteen attendances, five (42 per cent) had improved;

★ We felt that this was a reasonable index of the amount of treatment received since all the clinics used a standard period of time for each treatment session. We have not been able to allow for any differences in the quality or intensity of treatment received within such sessions and have assumed that all professional staff of clinics were equally proficient.

and, of the thirteen with more than fifteen attendances, eight (62 per cent) were rated as improved. Among the forty-one children who had never attended a clinic, 61 per cent had improved. Considering the situation from another viewpoint there was virtually no difference between the group who had improved and that which had deteriorated in respect of the mean number of visits paid to a clinic. The largest number of attendances had occurred among those children whose state was rated as 'unchanged'; they averaged fifteen sessions compared with nine for both the other groups.

The analysis so far has disregarded the possibility of variations in the severity of the children's original state. It might be argued, however, that the children who improved on minimal treatment consisted of those who were the least disturbed, and that those who failed to respond to more lengthy treatment were the most disturbed initially.

TABLE 46. *Outcome of children by initial rating of disturbance and frequency of attendance at a child guidance clinic or clinic-initiated class or school*

Original level of disturbance	*No. of attendances made at clinic or class*	Outcome			
		Improved		*Not improved*	
		No.	%	*No.*	%
'Mild'	None (controls)	14	67	7	33
	5 or fewer	3	75	1	25
	6 or more*	4	50	4	50
'Moderate'	None (controls)	9	53	8	47
	5 or fewer	6	75	2	25
	6 or more*	9	53	8	47
'Severe'	None (controls)	2	67	1	33
	5 or fewer	6	100	—	—
	6 or more*	2	67	1	33

* *This category includes all those attending classes and schools.*

For all grades of severity combined χ^2 *shows no significant association between number of attendances and outcomes* ($\chi^2 = 5{\cdot}25$: *d.f.* $= 2$: $0{\cdot}10 > P > 0{\cdot}05$).

The information detailed in table 46 does not support this contention. Eight out of nine of the clinic-attending children originally rated as 'severely disturbed' had improved by the time of follow-up, but only two of these had received more than five psychiatric sessions, and none had received treatment elsewhere, e.g. at a school for maladjusted children. Again, among the five originally 'mild' cases who failed to improve despite treatment, four had received more than five sessions of psychiatric treatment.

Table 46 also shows that there was no association between length of treatment and outcome at any levels of disturbance. In each case, the proportion rated as showing improvement was highest among those children who had attended for fewer than six sessions of psychiatric treatment. There was little difference between the rates of improvement among those children who had received no treatment at all and those who had attended on six or more occasions. In our investigation the number of children in any single category is too small for statistical treatment of the findings. These are, however, supported by those of other workers (Eisenberg 1958, Cytryn *et al.* 1960, Eisenberg 1961, Heinicke 1969) whose figures have indicated that improvement may result from short-term therapy in treating children with neurotic symptoms.

The present study does not, of course, touch on the effectiveness or ineffectiveness of long-term intensive therapy, since very few children could be regarded as having received anything of this type. Furthermore, the estimate of treatment has been based on the child's own attendances at a child guidance clinic or at a class for maladjusted children. Some advocates of child guidance would consider this too limiting, claiming that such work is with the family as a whole. Time spent by the parents with members of the clinic staff may serve a therapeutic purpose if it leads to a beneficial change in the family atmosphere but no attempt could be made to measure such indirect relationships in a study of this type.

It must also be emphasised that the clinic cases selected for inclusion were probably the least disturbed children, since psychosis and brain damage were excluded together with gross delinquency and other unmatchable problems. It might be maintained that the more disturbed children are the ones who benefit more from treatment. On the other hand, the children described here are typical of many of those seen at clinics throughout the country, so that a demonstration of the value of a small amount of psychiatric help or psychological help in such cases would be of some importance in a field where resources are so limited and waiting lists so long.

ENVIRONMENTAL FACTORS ASSOCIATED WITH PERSISTENCE OF DISTURBANCE

Since there was no ostensible difference in outcome between the treated and untreated children, it was possible to group them together in order to examine whether any of their family characteristics might be associated with persistence of disturbance.

a. *Socio-economic background* Whether or not the father's occupation was a manual one appeared to bear little relation to the persistence of disturbance: 68 per cent of children whose fathers were in non-manual occupations had improved compared with 61 per cent of those whose fathers were manual workers. There were, however, some differences within the working-class group: only nine (41 per cent) of the twenty-two children with fathers in semi-skilled or un-skilled jobs had improved, compared with twenty-seven (73 per cent) of the thirty-seven whose fathers were in skilled manual occupations.

b. *Size of family* The size of the family also seemed to be unrelated to outcome. The rate of improvement was 67 per cent both among the smallest families, with only one or two children, and among the largest, with five or more.

c. *Position in the family* The child's birth order in the family did show a significant association (for children with siblings, $\chi^2 = 7{\cdot}34$: d.f. $= 2$: $P<0{\cdot}05$) with improvement (see table 47).

TABLE 47. *Persistence of disturbance by ordinal position in family*

	Place in Family							
State at follow-up	*Oldest*		*Middle*		*Youngest*		*Only*	
	No.	%	*No.*	%	*No.*	%	*No.*	%
Better	27	77	15	58	7	41	6	67
Same	6	17	7	27	7	41	1	11
Worse	2	6	4	15	3	18	2	22
Total	35	100	26	100	17	100	9	100

Disturbance was most likely to persist among the last-born children, who were about half as likely to improve as were those who were the oldest of their family. Middle children were in an intermediate position with regard to improvement. This suggests that the presence of younger siblings may have led to temporary disturbances in behaviour, especially among children who were under eleven years of age at the time of the original interview (see table 48). In this age group four-fifths of the children who had younger siblings had improved two years later compared with fewer than one-third of those with none. It seems possible, therefore, that the pressure of the presence and activities of younger siblings could have been more connected with such temporary behaviour problems in

TABLE 48. *Persistence of disturbance at follow-up by age of child at*[1] *original interview and presence of younger siblings*[2]

Child's state at follow-up	Children aged 5–10 years[3] with younger siblings		no younger siblings		Children aged 11–15 years with younger siblings		no younger siblings	
	No.	%	No.	%	No.	%	No.	%
Better	23	82	4	31	19	59	8	62
Same or worse	5	18	9	69	13	41	5	38

1 *One boy who lived with his sister's family at the original interview and in a children's home at follow-up is not included here.*

2 *Including step-siblings in each case.*

3 *In this age group the difference is significant* ($\chi^2 = 7{\cdot}89$: *d.f.* $= 1$: $P < 0{\cdot}01$).

young school-age children than in adolescents. It is not unreasonable to see the young schoolchild as being under stress through the presence of younger siblings who monopolise their parents' attention and remain in possession of home and mother while he, or she, has to go to school.

d. *Mother's employment* Children whose mothers were working at the time of the follow-up showed slightly less tendency to have improved —52 per cent compared with 68 per cent of those who were not working.

TABLE 49. *Persistence of disturbance by changes in the mother's employment*

Child's state at follow-up	Comparison of employment at original and follow-up interviews: Not working on either occasion		Started working since original interview		Working on both occasions		Stopped working since original interview	
	No.	%	No.	%	No.	%	No.	%
Better	31	74	5	56	12	50	3	38
Same	8	19	3	333	8	33	2	25
Worse	3	7	1	11	4	17	3	38
Total	42		9		24		8	

A comparison of the mother's employment at both interviews showed that the highest improvement rate occurred among children when the mother was employed on neither occasion. On the whole, the children of mothers who were working at the time of the original interviews were less likely to have improved, whether or not the mother was still working, than were those whose mothers were unoccupied at that date ($\chi^2 = 3{\cdot}86$:

d.f. = 1: $P < 0.05$). The most persistent disturbance was found among children whose mothers had stopped working—probably because in most cases the return to full-time housewifery was a result of the child's increasing problems or reflected some other adverse event such as the necessity of tending a sick relative, the mother's re-marriage and pregnancy, death of the mother's employer, or deterioration of her own health.

e. Parents' health The parents' own physical and mental health seemed to have some bearing on the persistence of the child's disturbance. This was particularly true of the mother's health.

TABLE 50. *Persistence of disturbance by the mother's physical health at both original and follow-up interviews*

Child's state	Mother's health*							
	Good on both occasions		Bad on both occasions		Worse at follow-up		Better at follow-up	
	No.	%	No.	%	No.	%	No.	%
Better	30	67	6	40	6	55	10	77
Same or worse	15	33	9	60	5	45	3	23

* *The three children living in local authority children's homes are not included in tables regarding parental health.*

Table 50 shows clearly that where the mother continued to report that she, herself, was not in good health* the child's disturbance also persisted, whereas reported improvement in the mother's health was also accompanied by an improvement in the child's state.†

The majority of fathers were said to be in good health but, among those who were not, a similar pattern emerged. Once again, the highest rate of persistence (70 per cent) was found among the ten children whose fathers suffered from a health disorder, mild in all but two cases. In the six cases where the father's health was better at the follow-up, five of the children had also improved.

A reported improvement in the mother's mental health was associated with an improvement in the child's state also. Thus the children of the

* The ailments reported were mainly mild and included anaemia, bronchitis, miscellaneous aches and pains, minor gynaecological problems and two cases of 'blackouts' (possibly epileptic episodes), but one mother had undergone a partial gastrectomy and the removal of one kidney prior to the first interview.

† It must, of course, be stressed that these reports on health are based on the informant's own assessment.

twenty-three mothers who said their 'nerves' had improved at follow-up received an 'improved' rating in seventeen cases. Among the ten mothers who felt they were worse, on the other hand, only two children had improved. Where the mother complained of 'nerves' on both occasions, however, the children's improvement rate was fairly good in fifteen out of twenty-three cases (62 per cent), nearly the same as among the twenty-seven children whose mothers declared themselves free of 'nerves' on both occasions (67 per cent).

Reports on the mental state of the fathers changed less than those of the mothers. Only one of the originally 'healthy' fathers had developed 'nerves'; of the original sufferers sixteen remained unchanged, one deteriorated, one died, and four improved. This made it impossible to attempt any assessment of the association between changes in the condition of father and of child. Where the father remained unaffected by 'nerves', two-thirds of the children improved; where the father had persistent psychological problems, only half did so.

f. *Parents'* attitudes* When the parents had originally said that their primary reaction to their child's behaviour was one of irritation, the persistence rate of the child's disturbance was found to be significantly higher (55 per cent) than that (15 per cent) of the children whose parents had been predominantly worried and anxious ($\chi^2 = 10{\cdot}63$: d.f. $= 1$: $P<0.01$). Where parents viewed their child's problem as unavoidable, physical in origin, or non-existent, 69 per cent of the children were said to have improved, a close approximation to the overall rate for the whole group of children (63 per cent). The intensity of the parents' reactions was not related to changes in the child's state. Where the parents were 'very worried' initially, 83 per cent of children improved; among the 'mildly worried' 86 per cent. Similarly, 52 per cent of children improved when the parents were originally 'very irritated', compared with 47 per cent where they were 'mildly' so.

There was a marked association† between a child's failure to improve and reported stress in the family. Table 51 shows that the proportion of children with some conflict in their family was four times as great among those who had deteriorated as among those who were most improved.

g. *The school environment* So far, the discussion of the child's state at follow-up has been limited to factors in the home environment. In

* Children no longer resident with their parents were excluded from this analysis.

† For those who improved v. those who did not, $\chi^2=11{\cdot}27$: d.f.$=1$: $P<0{\cdot}001$.

TABLE 51. *Number of children showing poor family relationships by degree of improvement at follow-up*

Poor relationship existing	Child's state at follow-up: Definitely better No.	%	Slightly better No.	%	Same No.	%	Worse* No.	%
a. Between parents	2	11	5	14	5	24	3	27
b. Between mother (or stepmother) and child	1	5	6	17	8	38	3	27
c. Between father (or stepfather) and child	1	5	2	6	9	43	3	27
d. Between child and siblings	—	—	5	14	1	5	3	27
e. Number with some conflict	4	21	12	33	13	62	9	82
f. No apparent conflict	15	79	24	67	8	38	2	18
Total†	19		36		21		11	

* *All but one child came into the 'slightly worse' category.*

† *This is the total number of children in each group. The column total may be greater, as some children showed poor relationships of more than one sort.*

some cases, however, the parents specifically stated that they attributed improvement to changes connected with school. This was certainly true of the three children who had attended special classes for the maladjusted and also of a girl who had received remedial teaching for a reading disability. In all these cases, the benefit appeared to come from a very good relationship with the teacher concerned as well as from the actual class activities. Altogether, twelve of the children who improved were regarded by their parents to have done so after a move to a new school or class; such changes involved the loss of a disliked teacher or, more usually, removal to a lower, more appropriate standard of work. Eight other children, while remaining at the same school, had improved in behaviour and stability on achieving greater success or prestige at school. This was particularly true of children who had stayed on at secondary modern schools for an extra year in order to take some subjects for the General Certificate of Education (GCE), a process which transformed them into the élite of the school, enjoying more friendliness from the staff and respect from younger children. In all these cases, the parents thought that the child had greatly matured and gained a good deal of self-confidence. The other group which benefited was composed of four boys whose problems had involved 'dislike of going to school' but who had left by the time of follow-up: they had lost their anxieties and pains, and had settled down extremely well to work, even to the extent of attending day-release extension classes regularly. Only one boy had a poor work record: he not only disliked school but came from a very disturbed background.

Although based on a small group of cases, these findings add weight to those arising from the follow-up study of the deviant children. The results of both investigations strongly indicate that many behaviour disorders in children are transient and, in many cases, seem to represent reactions to environmental stress, resolving themselves with or without professional assistance.

Chapter Ten

Conclusions and implications

The work which we have described in preceding chapters was undertaken with the primary purpose of examining some of the issues relevant to the study of mental health and ill health in childhood. In this final chapter we bring together and discuss some of the main features of the investigation and their implications.

Our starting point was an attempt to acquire systematic information about certain items of behaviour of more than 6000 children, comprising a 10 per cent representative sample of the state school population aged between five and fifteen years in the county of Buckinghamshire. The items were chosen because of their bearing on children's mental health and the data were obtained by questionnaire. The more detailed information was provided by the parents, principally the mothers, whose reports have been shown by other workers to constitute a reasonably reliable source of data (Glidewell *et al.* 1963, Glidewell 1966). In our study the nature of the sample permits us to assume that any parental bias would be equally distributed among the various age-groups of the children; a useful internal check on validity was provided by the answers to questions about 'stomach pains' (figure 21, page 60) where the cluster of peak monthly frequency among pubertal girls manifestly corresponds to an indirect description of menstruation.

The first aim was to ascertain the distribution of these items of behaviour in a presumably normal population. Such information is closely bound up with the definition of the large, untidy rag-bag of 'behaviour disorders' which figure so prominently in the practice of child psychiatry. Since most forms of conduct which qualify for inclusion in this category can be exhibited by healthy children they cannot be regarded as symptomatic of emotional ill health without further qualifications; the age of a child, for example, is of manifest importance in assessing the possible significance of such phenomena as crying, temper-tantrums or bed-wetting. In consequence, the clinical significance of many types of children's behaviour may depend at least as much on how far it deviates from the average as on its intrinsic nature.

Obvious as it may now appear, the concept of morbidity implicit in this notion took much longer to permeate medical thinking than to influence workers in the fields of psychology and education. The difference in outlook was clearly expressed by Sully more than seventy years ago: 'Medical science is more familiar with the rare but striking cases of mental disease and defect; mental science, on the other hand, though it has learnt much from the suggestive analogies that may be drawn, has already shown that, during childhood at least, the vast majority of cases consist of deviations *within* the normal range rather than aberrations *from* the normal' (Sully 1892).

The early child psychiatrists were largely concerned with two objectives: first, the identification and treatment of brain-damaged and mentally subnormal children, and secondly, the study of pre-psychotic and pre-delinquent factors with a view to preventing mental illness in later life (Witmer 1940). The optimistic view of childhood as 'the golden age of mental hygiene' was quickly tempered by the experience obtained from child guidance clinics which made it clear that prevention was a chimaerical undertaking with the available methods. The organised practice of child psychiatry also established that children's behaviour disorders were widespread in occurrence and multiple in form, but none the less until recently the majority of clinicians were more preoccupied with the behaviour presented by their patients and its supposed psychopathology than with its relations with patterns of conduct in the population at large. In the past decade, however, the selective bias operating on those 'problem' children singled out for medical attention has been more generally acknowledged. Leo Kanner, the doyen of modern child psychiatrists, has drawn the appropriate conclusion (1957): 'This selectiveness, in the absence of "normal controls", has often resulted in a tendency to attribute to single behaviour items an exaggerated seriousness with regard to their intrinsic psycho-pathological significance. The seriousness becomes attached to the signal regardless of what it announces and who announces it. The high annoyance-threshold of many fond and fondly resourceful parents keeps away from clinics and out of the reach of statistics a multitude of early breath-holders, nail-biters, nose-pickers and casual masturbators who, largely because of this parental attitude, develop into reasonably happy and well-adjusted adults. But, in clinic statistics, those same symptoms, figuring among the traits found in the histories of "problem children", are apt to be given too prominent a place, far out of proportion to their role as every-day problems or near-problems of the everyday child.'

Inasmuch as this view points the way to the study of children's behaviour within the framework of a defined population of normal children it argues for the application of what has come to be called the epidemiological method of inquiry (Morris 1957). This approach to morbidity is of manifest value when illness is to be regarded in terms of statistical deviations from a norm rather than as an independent process. The history of medicine has provided several examples of this concept in the sphere of physical illness and, more recently, in mental disorders (Shepherd and Cooper 1964).

Since the unit of investigation for epidemiological study is the population rather than the individual it is understandable that there should have been obstacles in the way of this approach to the mental health and ill health of children. For many years psychiatry has been relatively well-documented in respect of in-patient statistics which have constituted a traditional source of data. By contrast, the child-guidance clinic is organised to deal with a predominantly out-patient population: reliable statistics are notoriously difficult to obtain about out-patients, and the coverage provided by child-guidance clinics has been incomplete in most of the geographical areas where they have been developed (Lurie 1969). A further difficulty resides in the necessarily indirect methods of data-collection in childhood. Wheras the adult is usually able to furnish indispensable facts about himself and his illness this is not true of young children. In addition, systematically direct observation of behaviour can only be made on very young children. It is not possible to study directly children in the later stages of development, since laboratory conditions and the presence of an observer would certainly interfere with the subjects' performances. Most of the relevant observations have therefore to be made by adult informants whose outlook and attitudes may influence the child's conduct (Mechanic 1964, Peterson *et al.* 1961) but who have ready access to the child during his daily life and can observe deviant behaviour.

As Cohen (1955) has emphasised, the view of certain forms of disease as deviations from normal rather than as independent entities has a long history in medicine. The application of this concept to the behaviour disorders of children, implying as it does the collection of a large body of normative data constitutes the basis of the epidemiological inquiry described in Chapter 3. The focus of this study was on the measurement of the distribution, frequency and intensity of reported behaviour in accordance with the view of Pringle and her colleagues (Pringle *et al.* 1966): 'The value of data gathered on a large group of children is that it provides workers in this field with a frame of reference, a "backcloth" against which to view the normality or deviance of behaviour manifested by an individual child, or a group of children, of this age.' The findings demonstrated the surprisingly high prevalence of many forms of reported behaviour which are widely regarded as symptomatic of mental ill health in children (figures 1 to 37). These data agree with those few studies which have been conducted on comparable lines and raise at once the two questions which have been posed by Lapouse and Monk (1958): 'Does the high prevalence of these behaviour characteristics, commonly considered indicative of psychopathology, signify that a large proportion of the children have psychiatric disorders? Or are these characteristics manifestations of developmental stress reactions occurring in essentially normal children?'

Clearly the first question cannot be answered in the affirmative since, as Kanner (1960) has pointed out in his discussion of the same issue, '. . . there is no absolute criterion for the normalcy of any of the common forms of behaviour problems of children'. With regard to the notion of 'developmental' reactions it is evident from the data presented in Chapter 4 that various forms of reported behaviour are associated with different ages. Some items, e.g. crying (figure 28), temper tantrums (figure 32) and fear of the dark (figure 3) diminish with age; others, e.g. stomach pains (figure 21) and nail-biting (figure 26) rise in frequency with the onset of adolescence. By contrast, other forms of behaviour, e.g. fear of people (figure 5) remained constant in reported frequency throughout the five to fifteen age-span. From the internal evidence provided by the figures in Chapter 4 it is also tempting to speculate on the possible associations between these age-linked items of behaviour. It is, for example, legitimate to suggest that the similar shapes of the curves for fears of the dark and animals (figures 3 and 4) differ from those for fears of people (figure 5) because the former phenomena represent relatively transient 'developmental' reactions, while the latter tap more stable attributes of 'temperament'. Or again, the remarkable similarity in shape of the curves for worrying (figure 36) and dislike of school (figure 8) suggest an understandable association for which some evidence can be adduced (Mitchell and Shepherd 1967).

It is imperative to acquire such descriptive data from representative populations if children's behaviour disorders are to be delineated. At the same time it is clear that the presence of a particular form of behaviour, even when recorded at an 'extreme' frequency or intensity, cannot be necessarily regarded as abnormal in a clinical sense. Lapouse (1965) has pointed out that abnormal behaviour in this context must be regarded as '. . . a function of two conditions: deviation from the prevailing norms in a population of children, and interference with function as measured by adjustment and performance'. We may consider these two conditions in turn.

As a working concept of 'deviant behaviour' it was decided that any item of behaviour which was reported to have occurred at an intensity or frequency characterising 10 per cent or fewer of either sex and any single age group would be deemed 'deviant' for that age and sex; if it occurred in more than 10 per cent of the children of a particular age and sex group, it would not be regarded as deviant. In the case of 'crying', for example, 25 per cent of six-year-old boys were recorded as crying at least two or three times a week compared with 1 per cent of boys of fourteen: crying was therefore regarded as deviant only in the latter case. It must be emphasised that no single cut-off point taken to indicate behavioural deviance can be accepted as definitive, any more than a single level of the systolic blood-pressure can be taken as the threshold of hypertension. Our object was to define a limited range of conduct to serve as an index of statistical normality, and it is interesting to note that Lapouse (1965) has moved independently towards a similar procedure in using the concept of deviance. Although her method of weighting the raw behaviour scores was quite different from our own she too accepted the 'highest extreme of the distribution of scores' as indicative of deviant conduct. While the cut-off point was fixed at 25 per cent because of the relatively small size of her sample, the results led to the conclusion that 'had the sample been large, a more constricted definition of deviation at the 5 or 10 per cent level would preferably have been used'.

Having obtained a deviance score for each item of behaviour we proceeded to add up the number of individually deviant items for each child in order to construct a total index of deviance. This score expresses for each child the number of types of behaviour which are atypical for his or her age and sex group. Crude as it may appear, the value of an 'additive' approach to symptomatology has been demonstrated by several workers. With physical disease, for example, combinations of symptoms have been taken to define chronic bronchitis (Medical Research Council 1966). For adult psychiatric disorders the 'symptom-count' method is implicit in screening instruments like the Cornell Medical Index (Goldberg 1969) and the method has been used for screening military recruits (Hunt *et al.* 1955). With regard to the measurement of children's behaviour disorders Douglas (1964) writes: 'A rough measure of disturbed behaviour is obtained by counting the number of symptoms reported by the mothers . . .' and he has scored each of a set of symptoms which suggested emotional maladjustment. Similarly, Glidewell *et al.* (1957) conclude: 'The more symptoms so reported (by the mother), the greater is the likelihood that the child will be round to be disturbed on clinical examination.'

With regard to the second condition, data regarding 'interference with function' have been derived from school observations by most workers who are concerned with children (Eysenck and Cookson 1969). At St Louis, for example, Glidewell and his colleagues (1960) who have studied the effectiveness of screening by means of a symptom inventory, have shown there to be '. . . a reliable and positive relationship between the number of symptoms reported by a child's mother and the degree of maladjustment reported by a child's teacher'. Chapter 6 includes a comparison between the data obtained from the parents and the teachers in Buckinghamshire. The findings demonstrate a significant degree of association between the occurrence of deviant behaviour at home and the reporting of problems of behaviour in school. For example, most children who did not exhibit deviant behaviour according to parental reports also belonged to the group which presented no problems at school. Further, deviant children were three times as likely to have had multiple problems recorded at school as were those who were deviance-free at home. On the other hand, it must be emphasised that the relations are by no means universal: thus more than a third of the children who were reported free of deviant behaviour at home exhibited at least one problem at school, and nearly half the small number of children with seven or more deviant items of behaviour reported at home by their parents were seemingly without problems at school.

Some such discordance is natural in view of the different fields of observation provided by home and school and the different frameworks of comparison for parents and teachers (Moore 1966, Rutter *et al.* 1970). The nature of both the overlap and the discrepancy is well illustrated by the findings of Rutter and Graham (1966) in their intensive study of ten- and eleven-year-old children resident on the Isle of Wight. Using specially constructed questionnaires which were given to parents and teachers they went on to carry out clinical assessments of children who were screened. They concluded: 'Both scales were equally effective in the selection of children with psychiatric disorder but to a considerable extent they selected *different* abnormal children.' In Buckinghamshire it was not feasible to make a systematic psychiatric assessment of more than a small sample of cases. However, it is noteworthy that a majority (80 per cent) of the children identified as attending the child guidance clinic were deviant in respect of their total symptom-score on the parents' questionnaire. In addition, the children who were matched with the clinic-attenders by virtue of their reported behavioural disturbances exhibited four or more deviant items in 74 per cent of cases; at interview the parents' description furnished behavioural profiles which indicated at least a moderate disturbance to independent assessors.

Since, therefore, there is some evidence to suggest that deviant conduct can be related to morbid behaviour the possible value of this approach as a screening technique naturally arises. Other workers (Glidewell *et al.* 1963) have discussed the problems of screening psychiatric illness in childhood in some detail. In part these problems reside in such technical questions as deciding on cut-off points to reduce mis-identification. There is, however, a more fundamental objection to be raised against the accuracy of any means of evaluating mental ill health in this age group on a single occasion: namely, that so many forms of children's behaviour may represent no more than transient reactions to short-lived troubles which barely qualify as emotional disturbances without further qualification. Our method of investigation precluded the possibility of assessing many relevant factors in the sample, and while our concept of deviance embraces the intensity, frequency and behavioural associations of an item of conduct it has nothing to say about duration. The importance of establishing the duration of abnormal behaviour is none the less closely bound up with the notion of illnesses; and if it be accepted that deviant conduct, however defined, *can* constitute a short-lived reaction to any of the numerous situations to which children are exposed, then it becomes vital to know whether such conduct remains constant over a period of time. It was for this reason that the follow-up studies were carried out.

Chapter 7 sets out in detail the outcome, in terms of reported behaviour, of two matched groups of 400 children, one originally characterised by at least four 'deviant' items, the other being deviance free. The 'deviant' children differed from the controls in other respects, including their family and social backgrounds, some aspects of their physical health, and associated forms of disordered conduct reported by both parents and teachers. In general, these children and their families emerged as less healthy and less successful; they were more exposed to stress at home and at school, than the control children. None the less, three years later approximately three quarters of the deviant group were reported as exhibiting a reduced number of deviant items, and about half were reported free of such behaviour. Parents recorded the same items of disordered behaviour in only one quarter of the group three years later; and, in general, the changes in pattern of extreme behaviour tended to follow developmental lines. It was not possible to establish any clear associations distinguishing those children whose deviant scores diminished with time from those whose scores remained unchanged.

Unlike this extensive, large-scale follow-up, the focus of the investigation summarised in chapters 8 and 9 consisted in an intensive study by interview of a much smaller group of children. These were regarded as being emotionally disturbed by virtue of their attendance at a child guidance clinic. Perhaps surprisingly, it was not found difficult to match the behavioural anomalies of these children with those of a group of supposedly normal children who differed from the patients primarily by virtue of the attitudes of their mothers. Here again, follow-up showed that nearly two-thirds of them improved markedly and, significantly, this was unrelated to treatment but was linked to environmental factors.

Taken together, then, the information collected over time indicates that behaviour suggestive of emotional ill health in children tends to recede spontaneously in response to developmental changes or life circumstances. Several workers have discussed the precise significance of the remission of what are often regarded as indices of emotional disturbance in children. Most have agreed that the disappearance of these phenomena can be used as a criterion of clinical improvement though Gardner (1953) has emphasised that this may not always be so. Our own data support the former view and since the persistence of deviant or morbid behaviour appears to be the exception rather than the rule we would suggest that the duration of disturbance must be taken into account when any item of behaviour be taken as a 'symptom' of emotional ill health.

The information presented in this investigation therefore leads us to conclude that for a large variety of children's behavioural items, it is necessary to take account of a number of factors before deciding that the item is, or is not, of clinical significance. These factors comprise *a*) the frequency or intensity of the item concerned; *b*) the 'deviance' of the item in relation to the norms for the child's age and sex; *c*) the presence or absence of other items of deviant behaviour, some of which may constitute a cluster, pattern or syndrome; *d*) the duration of the behaviour, especially with regard to its tendency to spontaneous remission; *e*) the attitude of the observer; and *f*) the circumstances in which the behaviour occurs. If, as we have suggested, much emotional ill health in children is more profitably considered in terms of deviant behaviour than of disease processes, then this approach should make it possible to outline the areas of conduct which signify ill health. Our own results express themselves in the form of associations with such factors as social class (Furman *et al.* 1965), separation, position in the family and medical history (Chapter 5).

The application of these findings to other settings must, of course, pay regard to the known variations in child-rearing practices which reflect differences in the culture and value judgments between communities. Many of the broader differences have been described by anthropologists (Whiting and Child 1953, Opler 1969), but a comparison of the behaviour of mothers and developmental milestones in five western European countries also indicates a wide spectrum of variation (Hindley, 1968) and, even within one urban community, class differences may be apparent (Newson and Newson 1963 and 1968, Stein and Susser 1967). The inclusion of such data into working concepts of morbidity is an important task for future research in which both clinical and epidemiological methods have their place. It may be expected to furnish much-needed information about causation and enable an accurate estimate of the size and nature of behaviour disorders to be made. Only then can provisions for services be worked out on a rational basis (Timms 1968). Davidson's (1961) comparison between European surveys of psychological disorders in children has made it clear from how many different standpoints this question is being tackled at present. Her conclusion that '15 to 16 per cent seem to need full investigation by the team of a child-guidance clinic' is a challenging but as yet unverified indication of community needs. It should act as a spur to the increasingly large number of workers interested in Sully's original, 'paedagogical' view of child guidance as 'the application of scientific methods to practical problems of treating, training and supervising the development of the individual child according to his individual needs'.

Appendix One

Inter-relations between behavioural items and symptoms

Previous work

The psychiatric literature contains very few empirical studies on the patterns of behavioural items or symptoms in children at different ages (Hewitt and Jenkins 1946). Such patterns of association could be of some theoretical importance. It is commonly assumed, for instance, that nail-biting, bed-wetting, thumb-sucking, and fear of the dark are all expressions of an underlying state of anxiety, though evidence for this proposition is lacking. Again, soiling is usually deemed a much more 'serious' symptom, than, say, nail-biting, but it has never been ascertained whether a child who soils himself is also more likely to suffer from a larger number of other symptoms.

The technique of factor analysis might be able to illuminate both these issues: how symptoms form patterns or clusters, and which are the more 'serious' ones. Factor analysis is based on correlation matrices, which could show clustering of items; the 'loading' might indicate the 'seriousness' or discriminative power of specific items. One of the few factor analytical studies of children's psychiatric symptoms which has so far been published was carried out by Himmelweit on the basis of data collected by Ackerson (1942) and is reported by Eysenck (1953). The correlations reported by Ackerson, on which the factor analysis was based, were for the most part low or very low, though they were based on 5000 cases. The factor analysis yielded two weak factors: a general factor of instability or neuroticism, and a bipolar factor of introversion/extraversion, which roughly corresponds to the division between behaviour disorders and disorders of moods and feeling, commonly adopted by clinicians. The patterns of associations were not very strong.

Very similar results were obtained by Oppenheim (unpublished) in two factor analyses of 404 cases collected by Grant and Grant at the Children's Department of the Maudsley Hospital. Between them the two factors accounted for 20 per cent of the variance. It should be pointed out that these studies were carried out on groups of children attending child guidance clinics where large numbers of symptoms are to be found, and not on groups of normal children where patterns of association might be weaker still. There are a number of well-known factor analytical studies by Cattell and Coan (1957), but these are more concerned with children's personality traits than with psychiatric symptoms. MacFarlane *et al.* (1954) report a number of weak intercorrelations between items and present five clusters based on twenty-three boys and forty-two girls.

Although the Buckinghamshire Child Survey was designed for other purposes, a number of attempts were made to study patterns of association between items of reported behaviour in the sample of children and to assess the significance of these patterns. The importance of the inquiry as a methodological exercise justifies the presentation of the results which were obtained.

Correlations

The most obvious way to obtain a measure of relationship between any two items of behaviour would be by calculating a correlation coefficient. There are, however, certain difficulties in this procedure. First of all it will be remembered that some of the items have been recorded on eight-point scales, and others on three-point scales. Consequently three kinds of scattergrams can be obtained: *a*) 8 × 8 distributions; *b*) 3 × 8 distributions; and *c*) 3 × 3 distributions. At first sight, product-moment correlation coefficients would seem applicable to the former, and Kendall's Rank Correlation coefficients to the latter two. Table 52 gives three examples of the process among the girls aged five to ten when the data are analysed in this way:

TABLE 52. *Correlations between pairs of behaviour items in girls aged 5–10 years*

(1)

Nail-biting	*Thumb-sucking* 0	1	2	3	4	5	6	7
0	773	11	2	7	1	4	21	138
1	30	3	2	0	0	0	0	10
2	17	0	0	0	0	0	0	3
3	16	0	0	0	0	0	0	3
4	15	0	1	1	0	0	0	4
5	35	1	0	0	0	0	2	17
6	53	2	1	2	0	1	3	16
7	117	0	0	1	1	4	3	32

Tau = ·091
r = ·093
normalised r = ·092

TABLE 52—*Continued*

(2)

Irritability	*Quarrelling* 0	1	2	3	4	5	6	7*
Phlegmatic	180	6	2	1	0	2	2	1
Irritable	861	78	32	24	13	22	8	2
Very irritable	89	11	8	3	6	6	8	9

Tau = ·178
r = ·205
normalised r = ·204

(3)

Food fads	*Appetite* Excessive	Medium	Low
Eats nearly everything	90	567	15
Definite food preferences	28	497	69
Rather fussy about food	6	121	200

Tau = ·462
r = ·505
normalised r = ·494

* *Figures 0 to 7 indicate the items recorded on an eight-point scale; 0 is the equivalent of* (*h*) *on the parents' questionnaire, 7 is the equivalent of* (a).

In addition to r and Tau, we also calculated r with normalised marginal distributions.★ This was done because in most cases the distributions were markedly skewed. As may be seen from these examples, the normalising process made very little difference to the correlations, but Tau tended to have a slightly smaller value than r. Strictly speaking, Tau coefficients would have been the most applicable to these kinds of tables but we had no computer programme available for these calculations, and moreover these coefficients are not suitable for the performance of factor analyses.

These examples also serve to illustrate certain other aspects of our material. It very commonly happens, as in the 8 × 8 table of thumb-sucking and nail-biting (table 52(1)) that more than half the cases lie in the zero cell for both distributions. One would expect this finding in a sample of 'normal' children, but it does not make for very high correlations. In the three-point scale examples the majority of cases tend to fall in the *middle* category. Altogether this whole enterprise is bedevilled by the fact that most 'symptoms'† are comparatively rare, occurring in only between 3 per cent and 7 per cent of our sample.

The size of these observed correlations is also quite striking; one

★ See M. G. Kendall and A. Stuart, *Advanced Theory of Statistics* (Charles Griffin 1967), vol. 2, pp. 567 and 573, examples 33·42 and 33·11.

† For the remainder of this Appendix, unless otherwise stated, the word 'symptom' refers to the third (extreme) category on the three-point scales, or to the top four categories (once a fortnight, or more often) in the case of the eight-point scales.

would have expected, on common-sense grounds, rather higher correlations between two alleged anxiety symptoms such as thumb-sucking and nail-biting. Even the correlation of 0·5 between food fads and excessive appetite is not very high. Similarly, there is a correlation of only 0·3 between restlessness in sleep, and nightmares. Thus the previous findings of weak inter-correlations are confirmed in this study.

Symptom cluster analysis

Exploratory analysis suggested that among children with five or more symptoms, certain items were more likely than others to be found together in the same child. Altogether, some symptoms tended to appear only as members of a cluster of four, five or more, whereas others might equally well occur in isolation, or might occur both in isolation and as part of a quartet or quintet. Two factors however made it difficult to proceed with this analysis: *a*) it was almost impossible to evaluate the statistical significance of our various combinations of triplets, quartets and quintets because the calculations of chance expectancies become extremely laborious; *b*) even with a group of, say, 1 500 cases the frequencies were very rapidly reduced to less than ten when specific symptom combinations of four or five at a time were sought.

All that remains, therefore, is the study of *pairs*, i.e. the joint occurrence of any two symptoms with a frequency which is significantly in excess of chance expectation. Table 53 overleaf shows such an analysis for all the symptoms of girls aged eleven.

This table contains only twenty out of the group of thirty-nine possible symptoms, namely those which were present more often with another symptom than would be expected by chance. The actual frequencies (out of 1 273 cases) are given in the lower left-hand part of the table, the calculated expected frequencies in the upper right-hand part. Bold frequencies are significantly above chance expectation.

Among the symptoms which showed very few significant associations with others were thumb-sucking, bed-wetting, tics, soiling, truanting, stealing, and reading difficulties. In this group, jealousy had most greater-than-chance associations with other symptoms, followed by quarrelling, sulking, worrying, headaches, complaining, mood swings and stomach pains. It must again be emphasised that these symptoms are comparatively rare in the sample, and that the analysis is based on necessarily small numbers.

TABLE 53. *Joint presence of pairs of symptoms, compared to chance expectations (girls aged 11–15; N = 1 273).*

		Crying	Restless sleep	Constipation	Temper tantrums	Complaining	Jealous	Stomach pains	Quarrels	Fear/dark	Worries	Underactive	Headaches	Nightmares	Sulking	Mood swings	Other problems	Dislike/school	Withdrawn	Lying	Vomiting
	N =	100	79	85	102	51	55	59	62	62	55	63	88	73	96	81	54	63	36	25	39
Crying	N = 100	—	6·2	6·7	8·0	4·0	4·3	4·6	4·9	4·9	4·3	4·9	6·9	5·7	7·5	6·4	4·2	4·9	2·8	2·0	3·1
Restless sleep	79	**12**	—	5·3	6·3	3·2	3·4	3·7	3·8	3·8	3·4	3·9	5·5	4·5	6·0	5·0	3·4	3·9	2·2	1·6	2·4
Constipation	85	9	**17**	—	6·8	3·4	3·7	3·9	4·1	4·1	3·7	4·2	5·9	4·9	6·4	5·4	3·6	4·2	2·4	1·7	2·6
Temper tantrums	102	**31**	**19**	**13**	—	4·1	4·4	4·7	5·0	5·0	4·4	5·1	7·1	5·8	7·7	6·5	4·3	5·1	2·9	2·0	3·1
Complaining	51	**17**	6	6	**25**	—	2·2	2·7	3·0	2·5	2·2	2·7	3·5	2·9	3·8	3·2	2·2	2·5	1·4	1·0	1·6
Jealous	55	**18**	**12**	**11**	**23**	**15**	—	2·5	2·7	2·7	2·4	2·8	3·8	3·2	4·1	3·4	2·3	2·8	1·6	1·1	1·7
Stomach pains	59	8	**11**	**19**	**13**	**6**	**9**	—	2·9	2·9	2·5	3·0	4·1	3·4	4·4	3·8	2·4	2·9	1·7	1·2	1·8
Quarrels	62	**17**	**9**	**38**	**23**	**7**	**18**	**11**	—	3·0	2·7	3·1	4·3	3·6	4·7	3·9	2·6	3·1	1·8	1·2	1·9
Fear/dark	62	6	**9**	**9**	**13**	**6**	**9**	4	**9**	—	2·7	3·1	4·3	3·6	4·7	3·9	2·6	3·1	1·8	1·2	1·9
Worries	55	**15**	4	**10**	**16**	**12**	**12**	**15**	**7**	6	—	2·7	3·8	3·2	4·1	3·4	2·3	2·8	1·6	1·1	1·7
Underactive	63	5	5	**8**	8	3	5	**6**	4	1	**7**	—	4·4	3·6	4·8	4·0	2·7	3·1	1·8	1·2	1·9
Headaches	88	**16**	**18**	**20**	**21**	**12**	**11**	**19**	**14**	**14**	**10**	**6**	—	5·0	6·6	5·6	3·7	4·4	2·5	1·7	2·7
Nightmares	73	**12**	**15**	**15**	**19**	**6**	**9**	**10**	**11**	**11**	**11**	5	**18**	—	5·5	4·7	3·1	3·6	2·1	1·4	2·2
Sulking	96	**34**	**16**	**16**	**33**	**19**	**16**	**13**	**22**	8	**12**	**9**	**20**	9	—	6·1	4·1	4·6	2·7	1·9	2·9
Mood swings	81	**18**	**10**	9	34	**18**	**21**	**8**	**15**	**8**	**13**	3	**14**	6	**28**	—	3·4	4·0	2·3	1·6	2·5
Other problems	54	4	5	6	10	**8**	**7**	3	**6**	**6**	4	3	4	6	**12**	**8**	—	2·7	1·5	1·1	1·7
Dislike school	63	4	3	7	14	**10**	**7**	5	**11**	4	**6**	**7**	8	7	**17**	**10**	4	—	1·8	1·2	1·9
Withdrawn	36	5	3	5	6	3	**5**	2	4	4	**12**	**6**	4	**4**	**8**	**7**	**7**	**6**	—	·707	1·1
Lying	25	**5**	0	1	7	**7**	**6**	1	**7**	1	1	4	2	**23**	**9**	**7**	**5**	**5**	1	—	·766
Vomiting	39	**9**	**8**	8	13	3	4	**9**	4	5	**5**	1	**10**	**12**	**14**	5	1	**6**	1	2	—

Scalogram analysis

In view of the obvious difficulties associated with the use of inter-correlations the possibilities of the Guttman-scaling technique (Guttman 1950) were also explored. This is one of several methods of attitude scaling employed to order respondents on an attitude continuum. The particular advantages of the Guttman technique are, first, that it ensures that only items which have *one* underlying common dimension are included; and secondly, that the individual's total score reveals which particular items he has endorsed, with a high degree of reproductibility, because the items are ranked. Guttman scaling can only be successful in a universe of content which will scale, i.e. one that possesses a considerable degree of structure and pattern and can be tapped by means of a unidimensional scale. During the second world war this technique was used to develop a six-item neuroticism scale as a screening device for the U.S. armed forces.

The Guttman scaling procedures are laborious and time-consuming even with the aid of punch card equipment. It frequently happens that a universe of content cannot be scaled successfully. At the best of times, one may have to discard about two-thirds of the items in the item pool. Even when results with a satisfactorily high coefficient of reproducibility are obtained, the scale which results often covers a much narrower range than the original item pool.

Since the patterning of symptoms tended to be relatively weak, it could not be expected that our data would yield the amount of structure required by a Guttman scale. However, as a first attempt we took 100 unselected cases from the group of boys aged eleven and over, and submitted them to the initial stages of scalogram analysis. One difficulty which arose immediately was that these procedures are not applicable when endorsement of the items concerned exceeds 80 per cent or is less than 20 per cent. It will be remembered that the majority of symptom frequencies in this study are of the order of 5 per cent to 7 per cent and that hardly any of them reached the 20 per cent level. It therefore became necessary to include the intermediate category (in the case of the three-point symptom scales) and position three and four (in the case of the eight-point scales). We were therefore no longer dealing with symptom categories as such, but with wider groupings which included such items of behaviour as 'a little afraid of some animals', 'tells an occasional fib', 'occasionally becomes cross', 'a little shy with strange children', 'occasionally seems lost in a dream world', and in some instances also the average category, e.g. 'about as destructive as most children', 'likes school about as much as most children', 'eats about as much as others of the same age'.

Once these intermediate categories were included, the item frequencies rose to much higher levels, and after the exclusion of twenty-one items with frequencies of either below 20 per cent or above 80 per cent an attempt was made to scale the remaining seventeen items. This attempt was surprisingly successful. For boys of eleven and over it yielded a Guttman scale of the following fourteen items, in order of highest to lowest frequency, with 90 per cent reproducibility: irritability; worrying; food fads; lying; not a quick reader; not keen on going to school; complaining; mood swings; jealousy; some fear of animals; headaches; wandering; shy with other children; withdrawn.

The fact that these items form a scale with a reasonably high reproducibility coefficient has a double significance. First, that the items have one underlying dimension in common. Secondly, that they have the cumulative ranked property of a Guttman scale: for example, a child who is jealous will also have positive responses recorded for 'mood swings', 'complains', 'dislikes school', 'reading difficulties', 'lies', 'food fads', 'worries', and 'irritability' but not for 'fear of animals', 'headaches', 'wandering tendencies', 'shyness with other children', and 'withdrawal'. Again it should be emphasised that each of these items includes both an extreme category and an intermediate or average category. The technique does not permit the construction of a Guttman scale consisting only of the extreme categories; but if each item be regarded as a continuum of behavioural frequency or intensity, rather like a character trait, then it is clear that some of these traits or behaviour characteristics have the cumulative properties of a Guttman scale.

The scaling procedures were next applied to the three other subgroups in our sample: boys aged five to eleven and girls aged five to eleven and eleven to fifteen. In each case the analysis yielded a Guttman scale with not less than nine items, and with not less than 87 per cent reproducibility. There is, as we shall see, a degree of overlap between the four scales, four items appearing in all four scales, and two more in three of the scales. This would seem to indicate that among the many forms of childhood behaviour selected there is a core of about a dozen which are *hierarchically* organized in such a way that can be predicted with reasonable certainty from the presence or absence of those items below it or above it on the scale.

It is important to repeat that, for technical reasons, the middle category on every item was merged with the deviant extreme. This means that in some cases the items on the scales should be regarded more as character traits or forms of behaviour than as symptoms. It may be possible in future to develop a new procedure which will use only the extreme categories. On the other hand, there are some items on which the middle category may indicate a mild degree of disturbance and it is best to consider the items in every scale on their merits, bearing also this point in mind.

TABLE 54. *Scalograms of behaviour items (from most severe to least severe)*

Older boys	*Younger boys*	*Older girls*	*Younger girls*
Some withdrawal	Occasional twitches or mannerisms	Some fear of animals	Occasionally restless sleep
Some shyness with strange children	Some temper tantrums	Occasional stomach pains	Somewhat destructive
Loitering or wandering	Occasional headaches	Some shyness with strange children	Some withdrawal
Occasional headaches	Taking things or stealing	Somewhat destructive	Some fear of the dark
Some fear of animals	A little afraid of new people	Occasional jealousy	Occasional crying
Occasional jealousy	Some withdrawal	Occasional worries	Not very fond of school
Occasional mood changes	Occasional mood swings	Occasional mood swings	Occasional worries
Complains	Occasional crying	Complains	Not a quick reader
Not fond of school	Occasional worries	Not a quick reader	Complains
Not a quick reader	Not fond of school	Occasional lies	
Tells occasional lies	Complains	Not very fond of school	
Food preferences or food fads	Not a quick reader		
Wories occasionally or more often			
Occasionally cross or irritable			

Each scale in table 54 has the 'worst' items at the top. The items have usually been worded in terms of their middle categories, or in terms of both the middle category and the extreme category. The reproducibility coefficients are, for each sub-group, 90 per cent, 88 per cent, 88 per cent and 87 per cent respectively, which is satisfactory for the purpose.

The following items appear *on all four scales*, usually near the less deviant end of the scale: 'complains', 'not fond of school', 'not a quick reader', 'occasional worries'. There are also two items which appear on three of the scales namely 'occasionally withdrawn' and 'occasional mood swings'. Four of the items appear only on the two scales for the older children: 'some fear of animals', 'some jealousy', 'occasional lies', 'some shyness with strange children'.

In sum, the analysis so far suggests that, among presumably normal schoolchildren, the patterning of deviant behaviour was virtually non-existent. The items certainly did not cluster in the tightly interdependent way that some theories would suggest. However, this finding is partly due to the fact that frankly morbid behaviour is comparatively rare in this sample of children. If the definition of a symptom be enlarged to include forms of behaviour which are unusual but not deviant, then the frequencies go up and we are able to arrange about a dozen items in each age/sex sub-group to form a Guttman scale, with the strictly ranked and cumulative properties that this implies. Not only does this procedure suggest a degree of patterning in the data; it also makes it possible to indicate, in each sub-group, the items of greater and lesser 'severity'. This problem will be taken up more fully in the next section.

The 'severity' of symptoms

Consideration of the degree to which each symptom forms part of a pattern with a few or with many others leads logically to the correlation of symptoms with the total deviance score. Since there is no external form of validation available one obvious way of determining the 'seriousness' of any type of behaviour at a defined age level for boys or for girls, is to find out how well it correlates with the total score, i.e. how well it predicts the presence of a greater or smaller number of other items of deviant behaviour, regardless of their nature.

Crude as it it, a simple count of the total number of deviant items attributed to a particular child has proved to be a useful discriminator between child guidance cases and 'normals' (see page 159). It would seem that such items are quantitatively linked to the notion of emotional disturbance whatever the quality of the items may be. With this in mind a total deviance score was constructed (see page 78) with which individual items of behaviour could be correlated. Clearly a high correlation might reasonably be taken to indicate some degree of disturbance; conversely, a low correlation with the total score can be regarded as being of little psychiatric significance. We therefore subdivided our cases by the size of their total score and calculated, for each of these groups, the percentage with particular items of behaviour. For example, with the younger boys (1876 cases under the age of eleven) the distributions were calculated for 'destructiveness', 'fear of the dark', 'bed-wetting', and 'nail-biting'.

The first two of these examples in table 55 show a close and regular relationship with the total deviance score, but the latter two seem to have, at best, an irregular relationship with it. At first sight, therefore, these might be taken to illustrate the way some items may be more severe than others. However, the more deviant items attributed to a child, the greater is the likelihood that he will exhibit any one particular form of behaviour,

TABLE 55. *Percentages of children recorded as showing selected types of behaviour by total deviance score*

		Total deviance score							
		0	1	2	3	4	5	6	7 and over
	N =	733	491	299	152	81	59	23	38
Behaviour reported by parents									
Destructiveness		0%	1%	2%	2%	1%	5%	13%	18%
Fear of the dark		0%	5%	13%	16%	28%	25%	26%	37%
Bed-wetting		0%	5%	10%	11%	19%	13%	17%	13%
Nail-biting		16%	18%	21%	24%	21%	20%	21%	32%

regardless of its nature. If, for example, a child has six deviant items, then it is obvious that the likelihood of any one form of behaviour being present is much greater than if the child had only one item. In other words, chance alone would yield a rising percentage curve with an increasing total deviance score, irrespective of the nature of the behaviour. Unfortunately, it was not possible to calculate how far the observed data departed from chance expectancies, taking into account the different frequencies of each of up to forty items for different age groups among boys and girls.

None the less, possible links between the total deviance score and any one symptom can be explored in a variety of ways. For instance, the means of the total deviance score could be calculated for cases with and without each item in turn. This calculation of pairs of means makes it possible to guard against 'false positives' by recalculating the mean total deviance score *minus* the symptom in question; this largely overcomes the objection raised above concerning the expected rise in the total deviance score.

The six items showing the largest differences for each sub-group are listed in table 56. As would be expected, these gradually change with age, and there are also some differences between boys and girls. 'Mood swings', 'worrying', 'complaining', 'temper tantrums', 'crying', 'sulking', 'quarrelling', 'jealousy', and 'stomach pains' all occur among the top six in at least three of our sub-groups. Overlap with the more deviant end of the scalograms in the preceding section is not great but there is almost complete agreement with the results for older girls set out in table 54. In fact, seven out of the ten items having the largest number of above-chance associations with other symptoms for older girls are also associated with the total deviance score.

There is one further finding to report under this heading. If the items are ranked in order of frequency of occurrence from high to low, and the rank of the mean total deviance score of children having a particular

TABLE 56. *Items showing the largest mean differences on the total symptom score, for each age and sex group*

5–7 years	*8–10 years*	*11–12 years*	*13–15 years*
	BOYS		
Mood swings	Mood swings	Mood swings	Mood swings
Worrying	Worrying	Dislike of school	Quarrelling
Lying	Sulking	Temper tantrums	Worrying
Crying	Quarrelling	Crying	Constipation
Complaining	Lying	Sulking	Obedience
Temper tantrums	Jealousy	Quarrelling	Stomach pains
	GIRLS		
Complaining	Complaining	Temper tantrums	Quarrelling
Mood swings	Mood swings	Complaining	Jealousy
Crying	Jealousy	Worrying	Complaining
Irritability	Crying	Mood swings	Sulking
Jealousy	Worrying	Quarrelling	Temper tantrums
Temper tantrums	Stomach pains	Sulking	Stomach pains

symptom is then calculated, a Rho-coefficient of $-0{\cdot}71$ is obtained. This indicates that the less commonly the item occurs, the more it is associated with other items. This bears out the suggestion that the more frequently reported items should be excluded from the calculation of the total deviance score; however, it does not make it possible to attach predictive significance to any one item.

Summary

As we have seen, it has proved difficult to find suitable ways of determining patterns, clusters or associations between symptoms. This is due partly to technical reasons, partly to the natural paucity of symptoms in a sample of normal children, but also due to the genuine weakness or absence of such patterns. Even in clinical samples, inter-correlations between symptoms have proved to be much lower than some theories would suggest. On the basis of these data it would not be possible to detect syndromes or nosological entities, suggestive of an underlying common determinant; further, the total number of items of deviant behaviour attributed to a child may often be more important than the nature of such items. It follows from this that the severity of any item of deviant behaviour might be assessed by the extent to which it is associated with other items of deviant conduct, i.e. with the total deviance score.

Appendix Two

Case histories of four matched pairs of clinic and control children

NOTES

To illustrate the matching procedure, the following usages have been adopted in recording the behaviour items listed on the questionnaire.

1. The main presenting symptoms of the clinic attender have been set in italics.

2. On any particular item when one child in a pair shows extreme behaviour and the other does not, the non-extreme behaviour is recorded in brackets. Where neither child shows extreme behaviour, the item is not recorded.

CASE COMPARISON 1

CLINIC CASE	MATCHED CHILD
Boy aged twelve years *Location of nearest clinic: same town*	*Boy aged thirteen years* *Location of nearest clinic: three miles from home*
ORIGINAL DATA	ORIGINAL DATA
Average rating of original state = 3 (moderate disturbance)	Average rating of original state = 3 (moderate disturbance)
FAMILY BACKGROUND	FAMILY BACKGROUND
a. *Father* Few details available; lived with the boy's mother, unmarried, for about nine years, apart from several temporary separations, but there was a permanent separation when the boy was seven years old; said to drink heavily.	*a.* *Father* Factory operative; aged thirty-nine years; 'slipped disc' otherwise good health; no 'nerves'.
b. *Mother* Part-time shop assistant; aged thirty-eight years; health good; very quick tem-	*b.* *Mother* Part-time domestic help; forty years; good health; no 'nerves' now but had been

CLINIC CASE

per, 'very nervous', worried a lot (see also d. below).

c. *Siblings*

Older half-sister: nineteen years (married and living in London).

Older half-sister: seventeen years (living in probation hostel).

Older sister: thirteen years.

Younger brother. eleven years.

d. *Other information*

The boy's mother had originally married a soldier during the war when she was eighteen. She had her two first children by him but had not had any contact with him since she and the children were evacuated from London towards the end of the war. She then met another man with whom she lived and by whom she had three children; this boy was the second child. He was not violent, as her husband had been, but he drank heavily and spent all his wages on drink. There were several separations and reconciliations culminating in a final split when the boy was about seven years old. The children were then taken into care (owing to the mother's 'debility') for about four months. This boy had also had previous separation experiences as he had been in hospital four times and had also been in care for one month at the age of one year when his brother was born. Shortly after his return to his mother, after she had separated from his father, he was again taken into care after appearing in Court as 'beyond control', and on this occasion remained in care for three years. During this period the only child to remain with the mother was the youngest. When the mother was given a council house, this boy (now aged eleven years) and his older sister rejoined her. The older half-sister was married by this time and living in her own home, though apparently on good terms with her mother. The younger half-sister re-joined the family for a short period

MATCHED CHILD

very 'nervous' when the boy was an infant.

c. *Siblings*

Younger sister: six years.

d. *Other information*

The mother had, herself, been brought up in an orphanage. The boy had never actually been separated from his parents but he had attended a day nursery from the age of two until he was four because his mother had become very 'nervous' and upset through coping with him in one room with a landlady who disliked noise and the father trying to sleep when he was on night shift.

CLINIC CASE

but was subsequently sent to a probation hostel at a distance. She had recently written to her mother complaining of 'noises in her head' and fears of 'going mad' (the letter was seen). The mother herself appeared very disturbed and told a story of persecution by *a*) an Irishman who had been showing sexual interest in her and who, on being rebuffed, threatened to break all her windows and 'get' her; *b*) his wife, 'a mad woman with staring eyes', who came into the shop where the mother worked and 'stood glaring at me for about five minutes without speaking'.

DATA FROM THE PARENTS' QUESTIONNAIRE

a. Medical problems underlined

No health problems; highly strung.

b. Hospital admissions

At six weeks: admitted for ten days: circumcision.

At nine months: admitted for fourteen days: scarlet fever.

At six years: admitted for seven days: observation for high temperature.

At seven years: admitted for three days: tonsils removed.

c. Behaviour items underlined

Very irritable, easily becomes cross or annoyed.

Has real temper tantrum, every day or almost every day.

Very destructive.

(Tells an occasional fib.)

(Will eat nearly anything.)

Always hungry, eats a great deal.

Very restless and fidgety, cannot sit still for a minute.

Tends to be very jealous.

(Loiters on the way home from school

MATCHED CHILD

DATA FROM THE PARENTS' QUESTIONNAIRE

a. Medical problems underlined

No health problems; highly strung.

b. Hospital admissions

No hospital admissions but was born six weeks prematurely and had to stay in hospital for eight to nine weeks after his birth.

c. Behaviour items underlined

Very irritable, easily becomes cross or annoyed.

Has real temper tantrum, every day or almost every day.

(About as destructive as most children of the same age.)

Tells deliberate untruths quite often.

Rather fussy about food, will eat only certain things.

(Eats about as much as others of the same age.)

Very restless and fidgety, cannot sit still for a minute.

Tends to be very jealous.

Wanders off for long distances or long

CLINIC CASE	MATCHED CHILD
or may go to play with friends without telling parents.)	periods without parents knowing where.
Usually resists when asked or told to do things.	Usually resists when asked or told to do things.
(Crying: no information.)	Cries every day or almost every day.
Bites nails every day or almost every day.	(Never bites nails.)
Has bitter quarrels with other children, every day or nearly every day.	(Never has bitter quarrels with other children.)
Has a very noticeable twitch of face or body, or mannerism, which takes place most of the time.	Has a very noticeable twitch of face or body, or mannerism, which takes place most of the time.
Moods very changeable.	(Runs on a very even keel.)
(Good reader, learned to read more quickly than other children.)	Seemed to have difficulty in learning to read.

CLINIC CASE: MOTHER'S DESCRIPTION OF THE CHILD'S PROBLEMS AT INTERVIEW

The boy was said to be very restless and quite unable to sit still for a minute. His mother's description of him sitting in a chair was of a person suffering from multiple tics, but this was probably an exaggeration. He had a 'frightful temper' and when he was angry threw things, including the furniture, round the room. He had recently broken a coffee table in the sitting-room by throwing something at it when he had been crossed. Once, when he was out with his sister, he had slipped off a stepping stone while crossing a stream and in his rage at this had lifted all the stones and thrown them about him. He fought with his brother and sister very frequently and had so terrorised his sister that she would sit on the stairs rather than go into the room where he was.

He was obsessional about shutting doors. If any door was open he had to go and shut it. The only exception was his bedroom door which he liked to be open at night. If anyone came into a room where he was sitting and shut the door, he would immediately go and check it by pushing it to see that it was shut tightly.

MATCHED CHILD: MOTHER'S DESCRIPTION OF THE CHILD'S PROBLEMS AT INTERVIEW

This boy was physically very healthy but had had breathing problems at birth. He was six weeks premature and for some time had to be fed by 'a tube through his nose'. He spent eight or nine weeks in hospital. Recently he again had 'trouble with his breathing'—made peculiar 'snuffing noises' and insisted on all the doors and windows being wide open.

When he was seven years old a tic developed. This started in his face, then moved to his arm, neck, shoulder and so on. Mother was very worried when it appeared and thought it might be St Vitus' Dance but once reassured ignored it and it disappeared after about four years.

He was 'very backward at school' and had great difficulty in learning to read. His parents were very worried about what was to happen to him in the future and had asked the school to give him homework to improve the standard of his studies. The school, however, had said that this was not a good idea. He had had a very good report in his first term at secondary modern school, but this latest report said he was 'poor in everything'. He seemed to

CLINIC CASE

He bit his nails very severely 'until his fingers bled'. At night when it was time for mother to come home from work he would stand at the window waiting for her to come into sight 'biting his nails'. He also kept calling to her when he was in bed at night—'I think he must hate me the way he gets me to go up to him in bed at night—as soon as I get down it starts again.' He was not affected by punishment, and 'laughs when I smack him'. 'He seems to like it. He says: "Go on, it don't hurt, do it again".' 'One day I think I will murder him.'

He had poor concentration and quickly lost interest in things. This affected his school work, as did the fact that he was easily embarrassed by having to read in class or being the focus of any attention. He was very careless and destructive with his possessions, according to his mother, but the examples she gave were of occasions when other people had caused damage to his clothes.

MATCHED CHILD

be very lacking in concentration and 'he just does not seem to care'.

He had frequently had temper tantrums in which he threw things around and lashed out at his younger sister. He was very defiant to his parents and only did what he was told if he felt like it 'otherwise he gets into a temper'. He never returned home punctually, for instance.

He was very jealous of his little sister and had resented her from birth. At that time he said that he did not want a girl, he wanted a brother, and ever since he has been unkind to her. When she was about two years old he shut her up in a dark cupboard. Since then she had been afraid of the dark and often in the winter he would tell her that he would put on a landing light for her and then run off and leave her in the dark. Two or three years before he had knocked her off her tricycle and during the last month he had kicked her on the way back from Sunday school and told her to say that she had hurt her leg by slipping off the pavement. He was very inclined to tell lies, often unnecessary ones. For instance, he travelled to school by bus and his parents bought him a two-monthly season ticket. Recently they had noticed that he often seemed to get very wet but he said that this happened while he was waiting for the bus. They then found out that he had been walking to school (about five miles) across the fields with a friend for about four months. This had been of no financial advantage to him as his parents had bought the ticket and he could not obtain a refund on it. During the entire period of four months he had told his parents that he had to leave home early so that he could get into his classroom at 8.30 a.m. and read a book. They had now found out from the headmaster that this was quite untrue.

He was always wanting his parents to give him things, but when he got them

CLINIC CASE	MATCHED CHILD
	seemed to take a dislike to them. For instance he had asked for a recorder for Christmas as they were going to learn to play at school. When he obtained it, however, he did not want it and had not even opened the box it came in. A neighbour had given him football boots which he said he wanted, but now he would not use them. Another neighbour gave him a geometry set as he was fond of making designs and 'he said he did not want the rotten thing' and gave it away to another boy. He had said on several occasions that he would like to leave home and run away and join the army when he was old enough. He told his mother that she preferred the little girl and was always doing things for her which she would not do for him. He was inclined 'to take things off other children'. He would bring these home saying he had been given them, but this was usually followed by a call from an irate parent saying that he had taken them by force and asking for their return. He was very fidgety and restless and inclined to 'roam around'. He had a habit of constantly tapping his fingers. He was very restless in bed and often talked in his sleep, discussing the day's doings and re-enacting conversations.
SCHOOL REPORT In a remedial class at secondary modern school; had temper tantrums; bit his nails; had difficulty in concentrating; 'an unhappy and sensitive boy'.	SCHOOL REPORT Attainment below average; usually near the bottom of the lowest of four streams at secondary modern school; restless; unco-operative in class; told lies; aggressive towards other children; at times he was interested and worked steadily but usually he was involved in mischief and trouble-making; very disobedient, always disobeying minor rules, showing off and focusing attention on himself.
FAMILY ATTITUDE TO THE CHILD'S PROBLEMS Mother seemed a very disturbed	FAMILY ATTITUDE TO THE CHILD'S PROBLEMS Mother complained about the boy for

CLINIC CASE

woman and her attitude to the boy and his behaviour appeared one of complete rejection and dislike (if not hatred). She could say nothing good of him and sneered at any kind remarks made by other people (e.g. his teachers or the clinic staff). All his activities were viewed as acts of deliberate provocation aimed at herself.

ACTION TAKEN

None except retaliation in kind by displays of temper and threats to 'get him sent away again' if he did not improve.

REASON FOR REFERRAL

The boy attended a very psychiatrically orientated school whose headmaster had originated the referral through the school medical officer. The parent would never have initiated referral and was unlikely, according to her own admission, to take advantage of the opportunity for help.

SITUATION AT FOLLOW-UP

Age: thirteen years.
Average improvement/deterioration rating = −1 (slightly worse)

CHANGES IN FAMILY BACKGROUND

The mother had remarried about nine months previously and, at the same time, the boy had been sent off to live with his oldest half-sister and her husband. He had not settled there and had run home on two or three occasions. On the last of these, about a month before, he had been ill with

MATCHED CHILD

the entire interview, for most of the time in his presence. She appeared to feel that the problems must have been due to her misconduct—'I must have made a mistake somewhere'—but had no idea how this had occurred or how it might be rectified. The main attitude to the boy and his problems appeared to be bewilderment; both parents did not know what to make of him.

ACTION TAKEN

These parents were conscientious people who were eager for advice and help. They discussed the boy's educational problems with the school (they attended all open days, etc.), but they had not been able to think of a suitable person with whom to discuss his general behaviour. They would, however, have welcomed an opportunity to do so.

REASON FOR NON-REFERRAL

In this case the school appeared to consider the problem one of naughtiness though, admittedly, school-initiated referrals were less encouraged in this area. The parents—although they would have been glad of advice—had no idea where this was available.

SITUATION AT FOLLOW-UP

Age: thirteen years
Average improvement/deterioration rating = −1 (slightly worse)

CHANGES IN FAMILY BACKGROUND

No changes.

CLINIC CASE

bronchitis when he arrived and was therefore remaining at home. Mother had become pregnant, to her great displeasure; she had asked her doctor to terminate the pregnancy but he had refused. Nevertheless she appeared more relaxed than previously. She had visited a psychiatric outpatient clinic in the interim, 'but they said there was nothing wrong with me'.

PROGRESS OF ORIGINAL PROBLEMS

The boy was still very irritable and had frequent temper upsets and tantrums; he was very destructive and at the time of the interview was at home instead of at school because his only coat and trousers had been covered with white paint. He was still very jealous of his siblings and appeared to be on bad terms both with his younger brother and his slightly older sister whom he still provoked a great deal. He was still very restless and 'all over the place'. He still bit his nails so badly that they bled. He still had very changeable moods and was extremely disobedient. He did not now appear to show the same persistent worry about all doors being securely shut, however, and would now sit in a room with the doors open. His relationship with his stepfather was far from good, although the mother felt that the stepfather had made almost super-human efforts to win him over. Within the last week there had been a particularly violent altercation between the boy and his stepfather. The boy had said that the stepfather had no business in the house and that he should not tell him what to do and, when told to wash before having his meal, had thrown the towel at his stepfather. The stepfather had then retired to sulk in the car for the rest of the evening, thereby 'humiliating' the mother, and had declared that he would now refuse to have anything to do with the boy or even discuss him. He felt, however,

MATCHED CHILD

PROGRESS OF ORIGINAL PROBLEMS

Mother said that the boy was still extremely difficult in many ways. His basic problem still seemed to be overpowering jealousy of his younger sister; he still showed aggressive conduct towards her and would punch, hit or persecute her on the slightest provocation. He still seemed to feel that his mother did things for his sister which she did not do for him though, the mother said, there was such a big age difference between them that this must happen sometimes, however much they tried to make things equal between the two. For instance, the boy had been cleaning his own shoes since he was nine, whereas his little sister (who was not yet nine) still had hers cleaned for her. He resented this strongly and the previous day had thrown his shoes down in the corner and said to his mother, 'You clean those! You clean hers.' On another occasion he had called his mother to come upstairs and bath him since she still bathed the little girl. He would also expect her to go up and find him clothes to wear even though the parents had bought him a chest of drawers and always put his clean clothes in it in a certain order so that he would know where they were. At Christmas time, or other occasions when presents were given, he would carefully count both his own and his sister's to make sure they had exactly the same number. 'Until very recently he would insist on getting into the bath with

CLINIC CASE

that 'something will have to be done, it can't go on like this'.

Mother said that the boy was perfectly all right when he was alone with her but became difficult as soon as anyone else tried to claim any of her attention. This was true, not only of her husband but also of the other children. He seemed to worry about her a great deal and always wanted to know where she was and what she was doing. Sometimes if she was in a different room or if she was in the house and he was outside, he would come frequently to peer through the door or window to make sure she was still there.

He never seemed to be satisfied or pleased by anything that was done for him. He seemed to be very immature for his age, though 'he is not mental by any means'; he spent a great deal of his time playing with his paper darts and little model cars and recently had started playing a lot with water. He would, for instance, put water into a plastic bottle which had originally contained deodorant powder belonging to his mother and then spend a long time 'just sitting squirting the water out of the bottle'. He had also filled an old talcum powder tin, belonging to his mother, with water and taken it up to his room at night. When he had been asked why he did this, he had said he had taken it to drink if he felt thirsty during the night; however, his mother thought this was a very odd reason as there were plenty of glasses in the house. He had also recently started to play with fire and to light paraffin lamps, in secret. On one occasion when his mother and stepfather had left him alone in the house while they went to the cinema, they came back to find that he had put paraffin into all the containers in the kitchen—'He had put it in the tea caddy, the salt cellar, and in all the glasses.' Such behaviour worried his mother a great deal as she was afraid that he might burn down the house.

MATCHED CHILD

her, so that he could make sure that she did not have any extra soap or water, I think.' The mother said this constant jealousy, which had existed ever since the sister was born, had so worn out herself and her husband that, on occasions, they wondered if it would have been better if they had never had the little girl and they certainly had not had a third child in case this would 'make her go the same way', though father would really have liked another member for the family.

The boy still had a violent temper and was aggressive towards other people. For instance, he had, on several occasions, hit his mother when she disagreed with him. He frequently hit his sister and recently he had broken his thumb at school hitting another boy. He had no sense of humour and if anyone teased him or joked at his expense he would retaliate with flying fists. He had grown a great deal during the last two years and from being a rather small puny boy was now apparently nearly as tall as his father, who was a large man. His aggressiveness seemed to be confined to people however; he was not destructive with his possessions and did not break things in his tempers.

He hated school, and had no interest in learning though the teachers at his present school had 'shown great understanding' and had been extremely helpful to him and to the parents. At one point he had wondered if he might stay on for an extra year; the headmaster said this might be a very good idea, as he felt that the extra year might bring out his potential. The boy, however, refused and said he did not want to 'stay at that place'. The parents wondered how he would get on at work if he tried to 'throw his weight around' and use physical violence as he did in his present environment. He also adopted an attitude of 'knowing it all' if his parents tried to explain something to him. For instance,

CLINIC CASE

MATCHED CHILD

recently he had wanted to do some repairs on his bicycle and had asked his father to help him. Once his father went outside, however, and started explaining about what should be done, he apparently took up the attitude that he knew much better and finished up 'shouting and yelling at his father' so that his father came in and left him to it. The mother said that the father was an extremely patient man and good with children, but even he felt quite often that he just did not know how to cope or what to do for the best with the boy. Recently three of the boy's friends who had left school had offered him the chance of taking over one of their paper rounds at ten shillings a week but he 'could not be bothered' and refused to take the opportunity.

He was still rather inclined to tell lies but was nothing like as bad as he had been. The mother attributed the improvement to the fact that most of his other lies had been detected and he realised that it was useless to try. He was said to be 'an outdoor boy', very healthy and liking to get away for long walks and outdoor pursuits by himself or with other boys. He was still very shy in the company of strange adults and if, for instance, the family had friends visiting he would sit completely dumb for the whole day apart from occasionally saying 'yes' or 'no'. This was true even if the visitors included children of roughly his own age. On the other hand, he went to the local Youth Club and had a dancing partner there but he did not see her at any other time. He enjoyed this Youth Club very much and 'seems to live for it the rest of the week'. He was still very resistant to parental requests. He had a very large appetite and would like to 'live on cake if he could'.

CLINIC CASE — SCHOOL REPORT

Not available as the boy had not yet returned to school in the area.

MATCHED CHILD — SCHOOL REPORT

Attainment below average for age; in the bottom 25 per cent of his teaching

CLINIC CASE

MATCHED CHILD

group; often told lies; very irritable; not interested in school work; immature in attitude to school; poor concentration.

FAMILY ATTITUDE

Mother was more relaxed generally and not so violently hostile to the boy as previously. She still rejected him, however, and was also very worried about the adverse effect which his behaviour might have on her present marriage. The step-father had accepted the other two children, who liked him, but was not prepared to put up with this boy, who did not. They were about to visit the child guidance clinic again in the hope that this might lead to the boy being found a place at a residential school.

FAMILY ATTITUDE

Both parents were considerably worried. They felt that the boy had 'thrown away his opportunities' at school and that this attitude together with his aggressiveness might make it difficult for him to be successful when he started work. They felt that the basic problem was jealousy but did not see what they could have done to prevent this. In general, they were still completely baffled by the boy and the best way to deal with him.

CASE COMPARISON 2

CLINIC CASE

Girl aged five years
Location of nearest clinic: nine miles from home

ORIGINAL DATA

Average rating of original state = 2 (mildly disturbed)

FAMILY BACKGROUND

a. Father

Technician; aged forty-one years; suffered from gastric ulcer necessitating special diet and 'arthritis'; tendency to worry unduly about his own health and that of the child and the possibility of accidents; also tended to worry about his work; first wife died, childless, two years after marriage.

b. Mother

Housewife; aged thirty-two years; physical health good; 'nerves very bad'

MATCHED CHILD

Girl aged five years
Location of nearest clinic: seven miles from home

ORIGINAL DATA

Average rating of original state = 2 (mildly disturbed)

FAMILY BACKGROUND

a. Father

Clerk; aged thirty-three years; health good; 'quick tempered' but also 'quickly over his temper'.

b. Mother

Housewife; aged thirty-three years; health good; very placid nature but once

CLINIC CASE

since the child's birth; spent most of the first year in tears because of loneliness following a move to a new area just before the birth, and difficulty in coping with the baby. She made her husband change the gas cooker for an electric one ('in case I put my head in the oven'); still found it difficult to cope with the child and the housework at time of interview; felt that her husband was unsympathetic and that her own siblings were uninterested in her problems and rejecting her—her parents were dead; tended to worry about child's health, e.g. any small scratch was bathed frequently in antiseptic.

c. *Siblings*
None.

DATA FROM THE QUESTIONNAIRE

a. *Medical problems underlined*
Travel sick; frequent colds or sore throats; persistent or troublesome cough; overweight; highly strung.

b. *Hospital admissions*
Nil.

c. *Behaviour items underlined*

Very restless and fidgety, cannot sit still for a minute.

Very irritable, easily becomes cross or annoyed.

Rather fussy about food, will eat only certain things.

Small appetite, inclined to pick at food.

Often seems worried, worries about many things.

Complains and whines a lot, hard to satisfy.

Has very noticeable twitch of face or body, or mannerism, which takes place most of the time.

Cries two or three times a week.

MATCHED CHILD

upset or angered tended to remain so for some time.

c. *Siblings*
Older sister: six years old; younger sister: two years old.

DATA FROM THE QUESTIONNAIRE

a. *Medical problems underlined*
None.

b. *Hospital admissions*
Nil.

c. *Behaviour items underlined*

Very restless and fidgety, cannot sit still for a minute.

Very irritable, easily becomes cross or annoyed.

Rather fussy about food, will eat only certain things.

Small appetite, inclined to pick at food.

Often seems worried, worries about many things.

Complains and whines a lot, hard to satisfy.

Has very noticeable twitch of face or body, or mannerism, which takes place most of the time.

Cries two or three times a week.

CLINIC CASE	MATCHED CHILD
(Seldom or never purposely destroys things.)	Very destructive.
(Seems a little uneasy unless a dim light is left on.)	Afraid of the dark when in bed at night.
(Seldom or never jealous.)	Tends to be very jealous.
(Seldom or never daydreams.)	Almost daily has times of being drawn into self and out of touch with other people.
(About as obedient as most children.)	Usually resists when asked or told to do things.
(Never sulks.)	Sulks two or three times a week.
(Never has temper tantrums.)	Has temper tantrums two or three times a week.
(Never sucks thumb or finger.)	Sucks thumb or finger two or three times a week.
(Never has bitter quarrels with other children.)	Has bitter quarrels with other children two or three times a week.
Other	*Other*
'*Until recently awoke every night moaning and crying for no apparent reason.*'	Nil.

MOTHER'S DESCRIPTION OF THE CHILD'S PROBLEMS AT INTERVIEW

The child was very energetic and demanding. Even as a baby she used to cry a lot and seemed to require very little sleep. When she was about a year old and learning to walk 'she had me walking her round the room for hours on end'. As she became more mobile, 'I had to run round the room after her every time I wanted to put a nappy on', and this still happened when she was being dressed to go out. At two years ten months she was sent to a private day nursery to give the mother a rest, but she did not settle there and was removed after a short while. When she was four years old, she was sent to nursery school. She then began 'talking and waving her arms about' in her sleep, 'reliving' school experiences. The mother took this as a sign that the teachers were not handling her properly and 'it made me feel upset and I started crying when I left her at school next day'. Mother also described an incident when the child soiled her pants at the

MOTHER'S DESCRIPTION OF THE CHILD'S PROBLEMS AT INTERVIEW

The mother thought this little girl was showing the effects of being a middle child, with only a small gap between herself and her older sister of whom she was very jealous. She wanted to do everything that her sister did 'and will not accept the fact that there are some things she can't do yet'. Both little girls had to be treated exactly alike—go to bed at the same time, have new clothes at the same time, etc., or 'there is an uproar'. She was very 'quick-tempered' and had real tantrums—throwing things, stamping her feet, etc.—but these were soon over; when she was younger she would bang her head on the wall when she was in a temper. If she were scolded or smacked she never cried but would go away and sulk for a few minutes and then return as if nothing had happened, 'quickly up and quickly down'.

When she started school she became very upset, clinging to the railings and refusing to enter the building. When she

CLINIC CASE

nursery and 'all the staff said she was naughty and stood around her looking cross'. Mother had said she was not naughty; the school lavatory floor was wet and she had always been told not to use a 'dirty' lavatory.

Until recently she would wake several times in the night calling for her mother. Now she woke only once—at about 3 a.m.—and asked for the pot. When her mother went to her the child insisted that she stayed and got into bed with her. If the father went instead, the child would settle down but, in the morning, would scold mother for not coming herself.

She had various fears; she was frightened of 'flames and fire'; of 'alligators and snakes'; she had to have a light at night and would not go to bed until father had come home; she would not go to the lavatory by herself; she was frightened of 'dying and going to Heaven'.

She was not encouraged to play with neighbouring children and did not like solitary games so that the mother had to play with her.

SCHOOL REPORT

Some loss of attendance (90/112) felt to be due to 'very slight medical reasons' and an over-fussy mother. Attainment average for age. In behaviour, she was restless and when speaking 'her words tumble out very fast'; she was also shy and appeared to worry more than other children.

MATCHED CHILD

was deposited forcibly in the classroom, there were tears until her mother left. Then, according to the teacher, she settled down. After about a week this behaviour stopped but when the next term started 'she had become used to staying home' in the holidays and ran home from school several times. 'I just put down what I was doing and put on my coat and took her straight back to school.' At this time 'her fear of school seemed to make her frightened generally' and she showed fear of dogs and some fear of strangers for a short while, though both fears had since disappeared. She also developed a facial tic but no medical advice was sought and this had also cleared up spontaneously.

She 'doesn't hear if you speak to her', but this seemed to indicate wilful disregard of the mother's requests.

She never talked about school and 'goes into her shell if you ask her'. Her mother thought she might be brighter than her sister but that she 'doesn't concentrate' at school and so was not doing as well as the older girl. The mother wondered if the disinclination to discuss school happenings was caused by the sister 'having gone through it all already'. The parents tried to show the same interest in school affairs as they did with the older girl but felt their efforts might lack spontaneity as 'it isn't new to us any more, we know what to expect'.

SCHOOL REPORT

Some loss of attendance caused by illness (116/136). Attainment average for age. No comments on behaviour.

CLINIC CASE

FAMILY ATTITUDE TO THE CHILD'S PROBLEMS

The *father* had arranged with the family's general practioner for child to be referred to the clinic for 'playing-up' the mother.

The *mother* fluctuated between denying the existence of problems and 'overloading' the child with symptoms—to show that she had, indeed, a great deal of trouble to cope with. She was very ambivalent about the visit; she did not want to be told about her inadequacy but did want a sympathetic ear for her problems. Her attitude throughout the interview changed from saying the child's behaviour was 'just her nature' to throwing the blame on to father's handling of the child and, finally, to a confession of her own feelings of inadequacy in coping with the problems.

ACTION TAKEN

Very little. Mother quite unable to cope. Father greeted on doorstep with details of day's disasters. General practitioner appears to have been seen fairly frequently but indicated that she was a 'fussy' mother and nothing was wrong—finally referred to child guidance clinic by locum G.P. at father's request.

REASON FOR REFERRAL

The child was being used as a presenting symptom of mother's malaise and need of help for her own problems. The immediate cause was the father's insistence on medical action to deal with situation in which the child's behaviour was being used as a weapon against him by the mother.

SITUATION AT FOLLOW-UP

Age: seven years
Average improvement/deterioration rating = -1 (slightly worse)

MATCHED CHILD

FAMILY ATTITUDE TO THE CHILD'S PROBLEMS

They felt that the child was 'going through a phase', which had been triggered off by starting school but which was passing over. They felt, also, that being a middle child had intrinsic dangers by inducing undue efforts to keep up with the older sister and to win extra attention by showing off. They felt that this was quite natural and that it was the parents' duty to provide the security and attention which was needed. They did not feel that there was any problem which would not pass away of its own accord without outside intervention.

ACTION TAKEN

Firm handling of the refusal to go to school. Other problems, e.g. the tic, were ignored but efforts were made to give extra attention and security to tide the child over the 'difficult phase'.

REASON FOR NON-REFERRAL

The mother thought that 'you ought to be able to cope with your children's problems yourself'. 'You should know for yourself what is going wrong' and then take appropriate action to deal with it.

SITUATION AT FOLLOW-UP

Age: seven years
Average improvement/deterioration rating = $+1$ (slightly better)

CLINIC CASE

CHANGES IN FAMILY BACKGROUND

A younger sister had been born eight weeks before the follow-up interview. Parental anxiety was also being demonstrated with regard to this child who was weighed before and after every feed to ensure adequate intake. The mother hoped the child would not 'turn out' like her sister.

PROGRESS OF ORIGINAL PROBLEMS

There was no apparent adverse reaction to the arrival of the new baby; the child appeared interested and pleased, and her mother felt she had to be prevented from handling the baby too much.

She still woke at night and called to her parents to go to her—the main reason now being that she was coughing and needed a drink. She had developed 'bronchitis' about twelve months previously and had been coughing and wheezing ever since. The mother had treated this with daily antibiotics for seven months until supplies were cut off. The child then coughed every night and coughed so loudly that it woke not only her parents but the next-door neighbours. She had recently shared a bed with her mother in order to enable the father to sleep in her room so that 'he would not be disturbed by the baby's feed'. The coughing had lessened since this happened. She wheezed a great deal during the day and her mother constantly called attention to her breathing by remarking on it. She had been shown breathing exercises to help her but she would not do them 'and you can't make her, can you?'

There had been some disturbance at school in the previous year when the child had had a teacher of whom she was frightened and at this time she developed a stammer. The teacher was said to have told the mother that the child was 'defiant' and

MATCHED CHILD

CHANGES IN FAMILY BACKGROUND

Nil.

PROGRESS OF ORIGINAL PROBLEMS

The mother felt that the girl had now passed through the rather difficult 'phase' that she went through when she started school. She now seemed to like school quite a lot and there was no difficulty about going. Problems arose if there were any change in routine or in staff. She became upset, for instance, if her teacher became ill and the class was taken by a relief teacher; she also took a little time to settle at the beginning of the school year when she encountered a new teacher. She was equally conservative at home and seemed to dislike changes in the family routine or even re-arrangement of the furniture. She was still inclined to be a poor eater and had a smaller appetite than the rest of the family. She was not, however, fussy about what she ate, and her mother said that they now realised that she had a small appetite and so gave her smaller helpings. She seemed to be very healthy and wiry, if a trifle thin. She still had a quick temper and was inclined to get cross rather easily. She did not sulk, however, and on the whole was said to have a 'nice nature'. There had been no return of the tic she had developed when she first started school, but within the last twelve months she had started to bite her nails. She did not do this sufficiently to make them bleed but they were, according to her mother, fairly well bitten down. She also sucked her thumb at night when she was going to sleep. Mother thought

CLINIC CASE	MATCHED CHILD
'would not answer questions'; the child had said she was too frightened to do so. The mother thought that the child's progress at school (particularly in reading) was too slow; 'she will be going into the junior school not able to read'. The school, however, described her as slightly above average in reading ability. She did not seem to have many friends and had recently come home complaining that the other children refused to play with her. She had also written a little story about a fir tree which was very unhappy because nobody loved it. She seemed to be afraid of being left alone—either in the dark or even in the daylight—if, for instance, her mother was in another room. On one occasion recently the mother had left her alone in the house while she went a message to the local shop; on her return the child seemed very agitated and upset. She was very restless in her sleep and recently had started either biting or picking her nails.	that she was 'inclined to be highly strung' in that she was easily upset by any 'telling off' at school. For instance, at the end of the previous week she had come home in tears because the temporary teacher had put her in the corner for laughing in class. This kind of incident always upset her. On the other hand, she did not appear to react unduly if reprimanded or even smacked by her mother. She was also inclined to be a 'worrier' and became very nervous about examinations and similar events. However, 'she seems to be able to overcome her nervousness' as she had come third in the last school tests and had recently taken her first ballet examination with honours, despite great nervousness beforehand in both cases. She no longer seemed to be frightened of anything, or to be at all withdrawn. She was still inclined to resist when asked to do things and 'always has to be told twice'; she always did them in the end, however ('I see to that'). There was still some mild jealousy and quarrelling between the three sisters, but nothing untoward.
SCHOOL REPORT	SCHOOL REPORT
Attendance good, attainment level above average; usually in the top 25 per cent of her class; worried more than other children; 'has a slight inferiority complex; mother worries over her progress and this may have been communicated to child'.	Attendance good; attainment level above average; usually in top 25 per cent of her class; no behaviour problems in school.
FAMILY ATTITUDE	FAMILY ATTITUDE
This was difficult to assess. On the surface mother showed anxiety and long-suffering acceptance, but the child's problems of health and behaviour were magnified even in front of the child, herself. For instance, reference was made to her 'poor reading' when, in fact, she showed better than average attainment. There was a strong impression that the	The mother felt that 'all children go through phases' when they required extra attention or reassurance for one reason or another. This child had gone through such a phase at the time of the original investigation and it had now passed. She would probably always have a tendency to nervousness and worrying but this was merely a part of her personality. So far as

CLINIC CASE	MATCHED CHILD
child's behaviour was used as a weapon against the father. Her 'bad nights' brought the mother into her bed (as did the arrival of the new baby) and her 'bronchitis' terrified him as he had a great fear of illness, especially of tuberculosis, the cause of his first wife's death.	behaviour was concerned 'a bit of common sense and a bit of patience' usually resulted in a resolution of the crisis.

CASE COMPARISON 3

CLINIC CASE	MATCHED CHILD
Boy aged ten years *Location of nearest clinic: same town*	*Boy aged eleven years* *Location of nearest clinic: eleven miles from home*
ORIGINAL DATA	ORIGINAL DATA
Average rating of original state = 3 (moderate disturbance)	Average rating of original state = 3 (moderate disturbance)
FAMILY BACKGROUND	FAMILY BACKGROUND
a. *Father* Moulder; aged thirty-nine years; physical health good; no history of 'nerves'.	*a.* *Father* Wood machinist; aged thirty-three years; physical health good; no history of 'nerves'.
b. *Mother* Left home when the boy was aged thirteen months, no subsequent contact with her husband or child. The boy was reared by the paternal grandparents until the death of his grandfather eighteen months before the interview took place.	*b.* *Mother* Separated from her husband when the boy was six years old but kept the children with her. When the boy was nine years old, she took an overdose of aspirin and, on discharge from hospital, went to Ireland without returning home or seeing the children. She subsequently remarried and returned to the area but her only contacts with the boy were accidental meetings.
Stepmother Married father four years before interview. Housewife; aged forty years; physical health good; 'very quick and active'; pronounced tic affecting both eyes; very tense; had been married previously and had son aged eighteen years.	*Stepmother* Married father eighteen months before the interview but had previously fostered the children for six months. Housewife; aged thirty-six years; developed a generalised psoriasis, except on her face and chest, shortly after her marriage; she felt this was

CLINIC CASE	MATCHED CHILD
	the result of 'boiling inwardly' with irritation at her stepsons' destructiveness and roughness; she said the psoriasis itched and made her irritable and unable to sleep; with social contacts limited she felt lonely. Had been deserted by her first husband on the birth of her second child.
c. Siblings None.	*c. Siblings* Younger brother: ten-years-old; Younger brother: eight-years-old.
d. Other members of the household Stepmother's son by her first marriage, aged eighteen years.	*d. Other members of the household* Stepmother's children by her first marriage: a boy aged fourteen years who was at residential school in term-time; a girl aged eleven years.
DATA FROM THE QUESTIONNAIRE	DATA FROM THE QUESTIONNAIRE
a. Medical problems underlined No current problems: informant (stepmother) had no information about previous illnesses.	*a. Medical problems underlined* No physical problems; highly strung.
b. Hospital admissions No information available.	*b. Hospital admissions* Nil.
c. Behaviour items underlined *Tells deliberate untruths quite often.* *Has stolen things on several occasions.*	*c. Behaviour items underlined* Tells deliberate untruths quite often. (Has helped himself to other people's things at least once or twice including taking things belonging to other members of the family.)
Very destructive.	(About as destructive as most children of the same age.)
Less active than average, likes sitting still as much as possible.	(About as active as most children of the same age.)
(Never restless in sleep.)	Restless in sleep every day or nearly every day.
Cries two to three times a week.	(Cries about once in two or three months.)
Sulks for hours on end about once every two weeks.	(Never sulks for hours on end.)
Bites nails every day or almost every day.	Bites nails two to three times a week.
(Never sucks thumb or finger.)	Sucks thumb or finger every day or almost every day.

CLINIC CASE	MATCHED CHILD
Has a very noticeable twitch of face or body, or mannerism, which takes place most of the time.	(Has occasional twitches or mannerisms which occur when tired, bored, etc.)
Seemed to have difficulty in learning to read.	Seemed to have difficulty in learning to read.

STEPMOTHER'S DESCRIPTION OF THE CHILD'S PROBLEMS AT INTERVIEW (CLINIC CASE)

This boy's mother left his father when the boy was thirteen months old. She was said to have gone to live with another man and had left the child with her own parents. The maternal grandparents said they were willing to keep him but suggested that his father should pay 'exorbitant' maintenance for this purpose. The father, who obtained custody during the divorce case, then removed the child to his own parents who were over sixty at the time. The boy lived with them until he was eight years old. The paternal grandfather then died and the grandmother, who was in poor health, felt that it would be difficult for her to bring up the boy on her own. He was therefore returned to his father, who had remarried about two years previously.

For some weeks the boy had been stealing biscuits at school break time, or at least taking them without paying for them. This was discovered by the headmaster, who wrote to the father to come and see him about 'a matter which he did not wish to put into writing'. The headmaster had already discussed the matter with the boy, who was repaying the cost of the biscuits at fourpence a week out of his pocket money. He had not mentioned anything about the affair at home. With a friend of the same age, he had also taken a bicycle which he found lying about in a wood. They took it to the friend's house and left it there and the friend's mother later came round to ask the family if they knew anything about a 'stolen bicycle'. He at first denied any knowledge of the bicycle but later told his father where he had found it

STEPMOTHER'S DESCRIPTION OF THE CHILD'S PROBLEMS AT INTERVIEW (MATCHED CHILD)

This boy's parents had parted when he was six years old and he and his brothers had remained with the mother until he was about nine. His mother then took an overdose of aspirin, rang up the police to tell them, and was admitted to a mental hospital from which she discharged herself ten days later. She did not come home but went to Ireland, where she married again. She had subsequently returned to the area where her family lived, but had not made any effort to contact her children. She had sent them Christmas presents, but they were not told from whom they had come. The children were apparently removed into care of the local authority when the mother was taken to hospital and subsequently were fostered, probably on a private basis, by the woman who later became their stepmother. She herself had two children from an earlier unsuccessful marriage but only one of these, a girl, was living at home; her son was at a residential school for maladjusted children and only returned for school holidays. She married this boy's father when the boy was ten years old and the entire family then moved back to the original house where the boys had lived with their own mother.

When the boys had first joined her as foster-children they were very difficult. Their behaviour was very rough; they swore; they were very destructive; and they showed uninhibited aggression. They were now said to be much better and this boy was no longer 'a real little savage'.

He had taken money which was left lying about. The stepmother often left

CLINIC CASE

in the middle of a wood and it was returned to the spot by the two fathers. It was apparently in a rather poor state of repair and might have been abandoned there.

The stepmother thought he was 'awfully deep'—'I can't get to him'. He showed no reaction to 'telling off' or punishment. This irritated her: 'I can't abide deep people.' She said that the school headmaster agreed with her about the boy's 'deepness'—this opinion was not substantiated.

The boy showed no overt emotion about anything. He was said to have shown no reaction to his grandfather's death or to leaving his grandmother 'and if he were told to pack up and go somewhere else tomorrow, he would be quite pleased'.

He had always told lies—'though brought up in a Christian home'. It was difficult to discover what form of lying was involved but it was described as 'silly lying'. The only examples given were of defensive lying when taxed with misdemeanours.

'He is retarded for his age.' He was very slow in his movements 'not lively like other boys of ten'. He preferred to spend his time 'making little drawings which I think are like a four-year-old's'. He took no part in any hobbies or constructive activities.

'He is always stuck in the house' and would not go out to Youth Organisations, etc. When he was not doing anything he would sit and pick at his nails and bite them. He also had a habit of 'twiddling his nose and sniffing'. He used to wet the bed but had stopped five months previously The stepmother felt that she had cured this by depriving him of all liquids in the evening. He was 'sulky'—no examples were given but he was said to go up to his own room and sit there sometimes. 'He is very destructive . . . If he has new toys, they are broken up next day.'

MATCHED CHILD

change lying on the table or the mantelpiece and had thought once or twice that some seemed to have disappeared. As everyone denied touching it, however, she thought she much have been mistaken. One day six shillings disappeared and shortly afterwards the boy produced a new torch. He denied taking the money and said he had bought the torch with his pocket money in Woolworths. The family checked and discovered that the particular torch was only on sale in another local shop where it cost seven and sixpence. As his pocket money was two shillings this made them almost sure that he had taken the money, though he continued to deny this. Nothing had been missing for about a year and the petty pilfering seemed to have stopped. The boy also lied, particularly to defend himself, if he had done something wrong. This was true of all the children who 'will swear blind they have not done something even if you know they have'. He used to swear alarmingly, but this had now stopped. Lately, he had become sulky and seemed to get in bad moods when he shouted at his brothers: 'Shut up or I'll bash you' and other such remarks. He did not show any outward aggression towards adults but his stepmother thought: 'It has been on the tip of his tongue to speak out at me once or twice lately.' He bit his nails frequently and also sucked his thumb. He found lessons at school difficult and had had some remedial teaching at his present school. His poor progress was probably partly due to very poor attendance in his early days. He had also disliked school originally, as he was teased and bullied because both he, himself, and his clothes tended to be dirty and unkempt. He was currently attending a junior school in the area where his stepmother had lived prior to her remarriage, and travelling there by train with her own daughter. He was, however, due to change to a secondary modern

CLINIC CASE | MATCHED CHILD

school in the near future, a move which would bring him back into the old area with the boys who had teased him when he was smaller; he was dreading this prospect.

When he had first gone to live with his stepmother he had wet the bed nightly. She had obtained pills from the family doctor and cut out his drinks before going to bed. He had tended to drink surreptitiously for a while, but had stopped when the reason for the ban was explained. He tended to try to hide his bed-wetting and used to make his bed and put his pyjamas to dry in the airing cupboard with the clean clothes. The stepmother had said that he did not need to hide his wet bed; he would not be punished for what he had done in his sleep as he could not help it. After about one year the enuresis cleared up and was infrequent. He had had a twitch of his cheek and eye, 'rather like a wink', as long as his stepmother had known him. This seemed to be getting worse. It was not referred to by the family and she thought that the boy was unaware that it was taking place. The other children in the family were not allowed to tease him about it but he might have been teased at school.

The boy had been very close to his real mother and had always thought that she would come back for him. Once since her return he had met her on a local bus, but she only asked him how he was getting on and gave him two shillings. After this he was 'impossible for two weeks' and no one knew what was wrong until someone else said that he had met his mother.

'He often sits with his mouth open when you are speaking to him' and looked as if he were not hearing a word.

SCHOOL REPORT (CLINIC CASE)

Regular attendance during previous term; his general attainment was below average but his reading ability was average; he was in the lower middle of his class; he

SCHOOL REPORT (MATCHED CHILD)

Regular attendance in previous term; general attainment and reading ability below average for age; in the bottom 25

CLINIC CASE

lied and had stolen in school; he constantly sought attention, and this made him a problem in class and produced difficulties in his interaction with the other children 'One of the most pathetic cases I have known in fifteen years of teaching . . . hated by his stepmother and regarded as the cause of matrimonial trouble by his father.'

FAMILY ATTITUDE TO THE CHILD'S PROBLEMS

The stepmother said that she and the boy's father were afraid that he 'would turn into a juvenile delinquent' and they didn't want a 'family scandal' over him. At first she suggested this was due to bad heredity from mother; later she changed and said in some ways he might 'take after his father'. The boy could do nothing right; when asked about specific items of behaviour, the stepmother, if she could not give an unfavourable response, would qualify her answer with 'but' and go on to describe some other item of behaviour which was a problem. She was very keen that 'something should be done' about the boy and showed great interest in residential schools. She said that she thought the boy's mother should have been made to take him back. Father was quoted at one point as saying there was too much fuss and the boy was all right.

ACTION TAKEN

Prohibitions, nagging, punishment—'thrashing does no good'. Father took the disciplinary action: 'He's his child so I leave that to him.'

REASON FOR REFERRAL

The headmaster at the boy's school, who was very worried about him, appeared

MATCHED CHILD

per cent of his class; sucks his thumb or fingers; has a noticeable twitch.

FAMILY ATTITUDE TO THE CHILD'S PROBLEMS

The stepmother found all three boys a strain to manage but thought this boy was the easiest of the three. She attibuted their difficulties to poor training in their younger days and to emotional problems resulting from their broken home. However, though intellectually able to understand the behaviour, in practice she often found herself feeling very tired and irritable. She felt that this boy and his younger brother would both benefit from residential school—as her own boy had done. This, of course, would limit the strain on her during term time and let her go back to her 'peaceful days' with only a quiet little girl at home, a situation to which she several times said that she looked back with longing. Her attitude to the boys, however, was kindly and though she was overwhelmed by the pressure of rearing three very 'difficult' little boys, she did not appear to reject them.

ACTION TAKEN

The stepmother was trying to 'train' the boys by example, reasoning, etc., and hoping that in time they would improve. Advice was also sought from school doctors in the hope of special school recommendation.

REASON FOR NON-REFERRAL

The stepmother's own son had been to child guidance but she did not feel that it

CLINIC CASE

to have exerted considerable pressure on the parents to get a referral to the clinic through their own family doctor—schools could not themselves refer children. Father thought it 'a lot of nonsense' but stepmother had obviously been motivated towards the clinic through hopes of getting the child removed from home.

SITUATION AT FOLLOW-UP

Age: twelve years
Average improvement/deterioration rating = +1 (slightly better)

CHANGES IN FAMILY BACKGROUND

The boy had been taken into the care of the local authority shortly after the original interview. He spent some months in a children's home until a place was found for him at a residential school for maladjusted children. His father and stepmother wished to have no further contact with him, so his holidays were spent in a small and relatively family-like children's home. The house-parents at the children's home also wrote to him during term time in place of his parents. The grandmother who had brought him up, but who was now very frail, also still kept in touch with him; she sent him parcels and letters while he was at school and had him to stay for a week or ten days in every holiday. Any further period would have caused strain on both sides, as the boy was active and 'usually grubby' and his grandmother was house-proud and fastidious.

MATCHED CHILD

could help in this case; the trouble went 'too far back' and was too deep-rooted in their early life with their own mother. She felt that, given time, she could train them herself and that a period at residential schools would be very beneficial. She did not, however, see the child guidance clinic as a way to achieve such a placement but preferred the school doctor.

SITUATION AT FOLLOW-UP

Age: thirteen years
Average improvement/deterioration rating = +1 (slightly better)

CHANGES IN FAMILY BACKGROUND

This boy and both his younger brothers were now all attending special schools for the educationally subnormal. This boy was a day pupil and still lived at home, but the two younger boys were in a residential school and only returned home for the holidays. The stepmother's son was also still away at school so that during term time the family consisted of the boy, his father, his stepmother and the stepmother's daughter, who was now attending technical school.

The stepmother's psoriasis was very severe and her own doctor had recently suggested that she should be seen by a psychiatrist. She was also sleeping very badly and was having trouble with her voice, which was very hoarse and 'keeps disappearing'. She had received treatment from a speech therapist but without success, as she was unable to relax or concentrate on the instructions given to her. She hated the holidays when the children were all at home because: 'I can't seem to get on with my work or clean the house properly.' She also felt that the skin flaking off from the psoriasis made the house dirty and she could not get it clean. She had been taking sedatives for about a year.

CLINIC CASE

MATCHED CHILD

The boy's mother had reappeared during the year and had called at the house to ask if he could stay with her for a few days. The boy said he did not want to go; mother wept on the doorstep and he locked himself in the lavatory for an hour and a half. Nevertheless, the stepmother felt that he was not unduly upset: 'Where there's no sense, there's no feeling and it doesn't affect him the way it would a clever, sensitive child.'

PROGRESS OF ORIGINAL PROBLEMS

In general, the house-parents felt that this boy showed no open problems of behaviour and was very easy to manage and well behaved compared to many of the children in their care. Yet there was 'something about him' which made him unattractive to those who met him. The other children in the home did not take to him, though he always tried his best to get on with them and was helpful and unaggressive. Nevertheless, when they heard that he was coming for a holiday there were 'groans all round'. The house-parents thought that there might be several reasons for this feeling, which they partly shared. The boys appearance was not attractive; he was rather deaf, possibly as a result of an earlier mastoid infection, and also had adenoids. He was a big boy, sturdy and 'barrel chested'. They were unable to explain exactly why, but nevertheless there was something in his appearance which was not attractive—'You would never look at him and say: "There's a lovely lad".' He was also a bit inclined to 'say silly things' when the other children were talking and would, on occasions, tell rather bragging fantastic tales to them. For instance, if they were discussing what they were going to do at woodwork, he was always going to do something very much better. The house-parents also wondered if the other children might resent the fact

PROGRESS OF ORIGINAL PROBLEMS

The stepmother said that there had been no trouble over the boys' recent stealing, which seemed to have stopped entirely. There had been one episode, however, about a year or eighteen months before, when the two younger boys had been brought home by the manager of the local supermarket because they had been caught taking sweets. They said that they had done this because this boy had told them that, since it was a self-service store, they could go in and help themselves. He was no longer quite such a liar as he had been, though he was still very evasive if called to ask for anything. He would now tend to tell part of the truth or to try to avoid answering, but would seldom tell a direct lie.

He was said to be becoming increasingly 'sulky' and to adopt a technique described by his stepmother as 'dumb insolence'. If, for instance, he was told to do something, he would do it but do it extremely slowly and provocatively and with 'a half smile on his face' which she found extremely irritating. He was also very sulky if he 'can't get all his own way', and on such occasions 'he will not speak to you for hours'. His reaction in general seemed to be one of simmering resentment rather than aggression. He was said to get on very well with the stepmother's daughter by her previous marriage, who

CLINIC CASE

that he stayed at home, since his school had a four-term year and, therefore, different holidays, while they went off to school. It was apparent, however, that these reasons were to some certain extent rationalisations, and the house-parents admitted that really they did not know quite why the boy was so unattractive. He was helpful, and would assist the other children and the house-parents and would also, when he was home, go round the village offering his help to gardeners the local farmers, or workmen working in the locality. He was very seldom in the house while he was staying with them, being an active outdoor boy. He did not like sitting still and even if he were watching television he could not concentrate for more than about ten minutes. He was usually quite purposefully active, however, and not just restless or fidgety. He was very fond of the dog who lived in the children's home and would take him out for walks. He did not, however, go out with the other children, mainly, it seemed, because the other children would not have him.

The house-parents did not think that he was what could be called 'a liar', but he was inclined to exaggerate events and present them in a favourable light. He was also a little inclined to daydream and they thought that he probably wove little fantasies with himself as the hero. He was not withdrawn, though his deafness, they felt, did sometimes mean that he was not quite in touch with what was going on about him and occasionally 'made silly remarks' as a result. They did not think that he stole, but he had a strong tendency to eat up any foodstuff or sweets that anyone else might leave about and, on his last holidays, had raided the larder on two occasions. Usually, however, he confined himself to gobbling up any sweet that another child might have left lying about—'Someone is going round saying "Where's

MATCHED CHILD

was the same age as himself, and to admire and emulate her brother when he came home on holidays. He did not, however, get on at all well with his own brothers. The stepmother said that she found this difficult to understand. She would have thought that, under the circumstances, he would wish to look after and protect the younger boys but, instead, he seemed to be very rough and unkind towards them. She thought, in general, that he was rather 'unkind' and hard in his reaction to physical suffering, but the examples she gave were very mild; for instance, he said 'serves her right' when a duck pecked a cat who had been about to pounce on a duckling. He also tended to laugh if one of the other children hurt themselves. He himself, however, did not stand up particularly well to physical pain. If smacked, he always cried and, on one occasion when he had cut his hand badly, he had fainted at the sight of his own blood.

He still sucked his thumb quite a lot and would sit sucking it and dreaming away sometimes for quite long periods; he also bit his nails. He also still took his teddy bear to bed with him. His bed-wetting had become infrequent and occurred always after occasions when there had been some emotional upset—either punishment at home or some difficulty at school. He did not appear to worry outwardly about these things, but the stepmother thought the bed-wetting might be an alternative reaction. The thing she objected to most was that he tended to hide the evidence when he had wet the bed. He had been told that no one would punish him for it. Nevertheless she continued to find that he hid his wet pyjamas under the pillow and pulled up his top bedding over the wet bed so that it would not be noticed. When taxed with doing this he tended to deny that he had wet the bed. He still had a tic in his eye and face, but this also was becoming

CLINIC CASE

my Easter egg?" and we look at M. and he has got a rim round his mouth.' Normally he had an extremely good appetite and was said to have 'hollow legs'. They did not consider that he was at all destructive; in fact, if anything, he was inclined to be rather possessive and careful of his belongings. In himself, however, he was inclined to do things which would get him dirty and dishevelled—'If there is muck around, he will find it.' He was always 'up a tree or down a hole' and this made him fairly hard on his clothes. They had not found him at all sulky, though they did think that his appearance and his deafness might make him look sulky when he really was not. He was normally obedient, but not excessively so. They had never seen him cry and they did not think he had any noticeable twitch or mannerism, though he still bit his nails.

MATCHED CHILD

more rare and seemed to appear only as a reaction to emotional stress of any kind. If, for instance, he had had a bad day at school, he would come home with his eye twitching. He still tended to go about with his mouth open and still seemed to have difficulty in hearing—or, at least, in reacting—when he was spoken to. He had had an audiometric test since he went to his present school and was then found to be fairly deaf in one ear. The stepmother was not sure how much of his failing to hear was due to deafness and how much to wilful disregard. She said it certainly seemed always to be when he was told to do something, or to stop doing something, that he failed to hear. He was a slow boy in most ways and not too keen on physical exercise apart from swimming. He liked carpentry or building models, and tended to become very bored when he was unable to carry out these pursuits. His reading was not good enough, for instance, to enable him to read a book and the family had no television.

SCHOOL REPORT

Attending a residential school for maladjusted boys; attainment average for his age; usually near the top of his teaching group, which consisted of only seven children; often told lies; had stolen on one or more occasions; very easily frightened; had a noticeable twitch of face or body; worried more than other children; 'a very insecure child; craving of attention or affection'.

SCHOOL REPORT

Attending special school for E.S.N. pupils; attendance good; attainment above average for the type of school; in the middle of his teaching group which contained boys up to two years older; 'has a most pleasant approach to and relations with staff'; 'a cheerful, merry boy'.

FAMILY ATTITUDE

His father and stepmother had broken off all contact with the boy when he was taken into care. His grandmother still took an interest, though in very frail health. The house-parents at the children's home tried to act as substitute parents, but were unable

FAMILY ATTITUDE

The father's attitude appeared to be completely accepting. The stepmother's attitude, however, appeared to be deteriorating. She felt that he was being 'difficult' and insolent towards her personally, and resented favourable comments made about

CLINIC CASE	MATCHED CHILD
to feel the warmth towards him that they would have wished.	him by other people such as his headmaster. She found boys difficult to understand and longed for the days when there were only herself and her daughter. She was irritated by 'slow easy-going people' such as the boy and, by implication, his father.

CASE COMPARISON 4

CLINIC CASE	MATCHED CHILD
Girl aged six years *Location of nearest clinic: six miles from home*	*Girl aged seven years* *Location of nearest clinic: same town*
ORIGINAL DATA	ORIGINAL DATA
Average rating of original state = 4 (severe disturbance)	Average rating of original state = 3 (moderate disturbance)
FAMILY BACKGROUND	FAMILY BACKGROUND
a. *Father* Factory machinist; aged thirty-three years; gastric ulcer; no history of 'nerves'.	*a.* *Father* Felting machine operator; aged thirty-eight years; suffered from migraine and bad nose bleeding; very easily upset, e.g. cried when child had asthma attack; vomited when children quarrelled too much.
b. *Mother* Housewife; aged thirty years; physical health good; worried a lot, easily became 'worked up'; had wanted a boy and was disappointed when her first two children were both girls.	*b.* *Mother* Housewife; aged twenty-eight years; overweight, asthmatic as a child; 'nerves very bad' for previous two years; very irritable; at one time could not bear to be alone in the house; receiving treatment from the general practitioner who had suggested psychiatric referral, which frightened her a great deal so that she refused. She had not wanted any children; they were all 'accidents', but she would have preferred a boy when this girl was born.
c. *Siblings* Older sister: eight years. Younger brother: five years. Younger sister: two and a half years.	*c.* *Siblings* Older sister: eight years. Younger brother: five years.

CLINIC CASE	MATCHED CHILD
DATA FROM THE PARENTS' QUESTIONNAIRE	DATA FROM THE PARENTS' QUESTIONNAIRE
a. *Medical problems underlined*	*a.* *Medical problems underlined*
Travel sick; persistent and troublesome cough; suffered from skin trouble which lasted for two weeks or longer; eczema; asthma; highly strung.	Suffered from skin trouble which lasted for two weeks or longer; asthma; eczema; highly strung.
b. *Hospital admissions*	*b.* *Hospital admissions*
At five years: admitted for four weeks because of eczema.	Nil.
c. *Behaviour items underlined*	*c.* *Behaviour items underlined*
(*Eczema* (see *a* above) was the main referral problem.)	
Afraid of the dark when in bed at night.	(Seems a little uneasy unless a dim light is left on.)
Tells deliberate untruths quite often.	(Tells an occasional fib.)
Dislikes going to school.	(Likes school as much as most children.)
Very irritable, easily becomes cross or annoyed.	(Occasionally becomes cross—for instance, if tired or provoked by other children.)
Rather fussy about food, will eat only certain things.	Rather fussy about food, will eat only certain things.
Small appetite, inclined to pick at food.	Small appetite, inclined to pick at food.
Complains and whines a lot, hard to satisfy.	(Complains about as much as most children of the same age.)
Very restless and fidgety, cannot sit still for a minute.	(About as active as most children of the same age.)
Tends to be very jealous.	(Seldom or never jealous.)
Usually resists when asked or told to do things.	(About as obedient as most children.)
Moods very changeable, on top of the world one minute, down the next for no particular reason.	(Occasional changes of mood in response to things that happen.)
Unpleasant dreams every day or almost every day.	Unpleasant dreams about once a month.
(Is never restless in sleep.)	Restless in sleep every day or almost every day.
Vomits two or three times a week, as a result of coughing.	(Never vomits.)
Cries every day or almost every day.	Cries two or three times a week.
Sulks two or three times a week.	(Never sulks.)

CLINIC CASE

Has temper tantrums, two or three times a week.

Sucks thumb every day.

Has bitter quarrels with other children two or three times a week.

MOTHER'S DESCRIPTION OF THE CHILD'S PROBLEMS AT INTERVIEW

The child had very severe eczema and exacerbated it by scratching so that her clothes had to be boiled every day and her bed-clothes about every second day.

She also had attacks of coughing which continued for up to two hours—'they go on until she is sick and brings up phlegm'. These attacks happened quite frequently—for instance, twice in the previous week—and occurred if she didn't want to go to school or 'if she had been hurrying'. The example given involved 'hurrying' to put right a mistake which the child had made in running a message for her mother and for which she had been scolded.

She did not like school and said that she had aches and pains 'to get out of going'. She would say that she could not eat lunch because she felt sick and, if offered the choice of bed or school, would prefer to go to bed. If sent to school 'she will go down the street crying'. She 'seemed to like' being vaguely ill and often asked for an aspirin, which she was not given, for a 'headache' or 'stomach-ache'.

She was very easily upset; for instance, if told to do anything or teased by her siblings 'she will burst out crying'. She did not cry in the usual way but 'in a sort of whine'.

She was very jealous of her older sister and younger brother and 'always thinks they are getting a better deal than she is'. She bitterly resented the fact that her older sister was born in France, when her father was in the army, and that she always got new clothes because there was no older

MATCHED CHILD

(Never has temper tantrums.)

Sucks thumb every day.

(Never has bitter quarrels with other children.)

MOTHER'S DESCRIPTION OF THE CHILD'S PROBLEMS AT INTERVIEW

She developed eczema when she was about six months old, though, even previously, she had some 'skin trouble' behind her ears. She had had eczema ever since on and off, mainly behind her knees and inside her elbows.

She developed asthma when she was eighteen months old, although this was initially believed to be bronchitis. She got very 'worked up' about her asthma attacks. 'She starts screaming as soon as the wheezing starts and cries out: "Oh Mummy! Mummy! don't let me cough; send for the doctor; send me to hospital".' Mother, herself, had asthma until the age of seven years.

She complained frequently of headaches, as did her older sister. Her mother thought that these were inherited from the father, who suffered badly from migraine—'people like us shouldn't have children, bringing them into the world just to suffer'.

She argued constantly with her sister and brother, but mainly with her sister because they shared a bedroom and argued in bed. This upset the father, who had been brought up never to argue or fight with his brothers. For instance, on the morning of the interview the father had been so upset by the girls' arguing that he vomited after breakfast.

She was faddy about food, but not so much now as when she was younger. She was not keen on green vegetables, but would eat some occasionally 'to please me if I have been cross about something'.

Sometimes she said she did not like

CLINIC CASE

child to hand them down to her. All the children received some new clothes of their own in strict rotation as funds became available. She was also very resentful that her younger brother did not go to school until after his fifth birthday whereas she had to go before: this was due to the administration of the local school, not parental choice.

She often lied and said she had not done something 'really and truly' when, in fact, she had done it. She would also accuse one of the other children and sometimes, weeks later, would admit that she, herself, was the culprit.

She had 'frightful tempers', usually directed at her brother, in which she shouted and threw herself about.

When playing games with her brother and sister, she often cheated and 'sweeps the pieces off the board'. Then, when they refused to let her play with them she 'whines about it for hours'. She would not go out to play with the other children, but preferred staying in with adults and was especially happy if she could sit on her father's or uncle's knee.

In bed at night she was very frightened of the dark and, even if she were asleep, would wake up screaming if the light went off. She made a crying and whining sound in her sleep and sometimes had to be lifted out of bed twice during the night to wake her and stop this. When she woke she had no recollection of the dream or what had been upsetting her.

SCHOOL REPORT

Attainment average for age; usually in the middle 50 per cent of her teaching group; behaved 'pretty normally' in school; wanted slightly more attention than average, but no more than many others.

MATCHED CHILD

school meals, and the mother wondered if she 'ought to send a note'; she at other times thought they were 'smashing'. She told lies frequently: 'all the children tell lies and I think it is awful; I never told lies as a child. I was heartbroken when my children first told me a lie.' Her lying was mainly defensive, 'though I always tell them that they won't be punished if they own up'.

She sucked her thumb very frequently and liked to tickle her nose at the same time with an old frayed piece of blanket. This had to be taken with her if she went out—for instance, to the cinema—and was taken to bed with her at night.

She often seemed to 'sit and let the world go by' sucking her thumb, particularly on the day before an asthma attack.

For a year when she first started school, she would not go into the classroom unless her mother went with her and the teacher came to meet her and took her hand also. If she was left at the school gates she 'made terrible scenes' and turned and followed her mother home again. At first the mother thought it was 'a battle of wits', shouting at the child, dragging her bodily and 'sometimes I've given her a good hiding in the street', but then decided 'I had better go easy with her—what with her being an asthmatic'.

Mother was suffering from her own 'nerves' at this time—'often I could hardly drag myself from the bed'—and the school had suggested this might be the root of the trouble; however, the mother could not accept this idea.

SCHOOL REPORT

Attainment average for age; usually in the middle 50 per cent of her teaching group; sucked her thumb; worried more than other children; had on one or more occasions shown tears on arrival or refusal to come into the school building, but this

CLINIC CASE

FAMILY ATTITUDE TO THE CHILD'S PROBLEMS

They felt anxious and unable to cope—'sometimes you just don't know what to do; you don't seem to be able to do anything with her'. The mother tried to be fair and patient, but found her constant whining and crying 'getting on my nerves'; in consequence, she became irritable and impatient, though she realised this aggravated matters.

She also felt resentful of the damage to clothes and bed-clothes caused by contact with eczema which had been scratched and the resultant necessity to boil them nearly every day.

ACTION TAKEN

Medical advice was sought for the eczema and the asthma, from both a general practitioner and a paediatrician. The mother tried to cope with behaviour problems by encouragement, punishment, reasoning and explanation.

REASON FOR REFERRAL

The child's eczema had brought her into contact with a paediatrician who worked in close co-operation with the local child guidance clinic and arranged for the child to be treated there. This

MATCHED CHILD

was felt to be 'more of a mother complex than fear of school'.

FAMILY ATTITUDE TO THE CHILD'S PROBLEMS

Father tended to become rather upset and frightened by the asthma attacks. Mother's attitude was a much more complex mixture of resentment and a compensating wish to magnify the importance of 'being asthmatic'. Thus, she admitted that the little girl's cough 'gets on my nerves' and that she had told her to 'try and stop it'. When, however, the child said her teacher had told her not to cough in class, her mother's immediate response was to tell her 'I'm going to write a note to Miss —— to tell her it's an asthma cough'.

The maternal grandmother was quoted as saying that the little girl was inclined to over-dramatise herself and her symptoms. Mother had also wondered 'if she couldn't help herself more', but immediately followed this opinion with 'but, of course she can't help it, it's not her fault—she's only a little girl'.

The child came home for lunch at the end of the interview and was greeted: 'How are you? Have you wheezed this morning?'

ACTION TAKEN

Medical advice was constantly sought on health problems from the family doctor. Behaviour problems, e.g. school refusal, were met by a mixture of irritation—slaps—and over-protectiveness—notes to school and insistence on recognition of, and allowance for, the existence of the child's asthma.

REASON FOR NON-REFERRAL

The child's asthma and eczema were being treated on a purely physical basis by the family doctor. Mother thought child guidance clinics were for 'mental or very troublesome children' and, in general,

CLINIC CASE

opportunity was willingly accepted by the parents, who felt that they were in need of professional help.

SITUATION AT FOLLOW-UP

Age: eight years
Average improvement/deterioration rating = 0 (the same)

CHANGES IN FAMILY BACKGROUND

A baby brother had been born seven months previously. The father had been in poor health; he had been off work for three weeks with a 'thrombosis in his leg' and had been put on a diet to lose weight. This had aggravated his gastric ulcer. The mother was on poor terms with her in-laws, who, she felt, 'looked down' on her and thought she had too many children. 'They think it's indecent because they've only got one or two.'

PROGRESS OF ORIGINAL PROBLEMS

The asthma was said to be very much better and, although the child was 'wheezy' most of the time, she did not often have a full-scale attack. The eczema had also cleared up shortly after her seventh birthday, but had reappeared after the birth of her youngest brother, now aged seven months, and had become fairly widespread. The family were carrying out a deliberate

MATCHED CHILD

seemed to have some fear of psychiatry; the general practitioner's suggestion that she, herself, should be seen at a psychiatric out-patient clinic was greeted with 'If you do that to me, Doctor, I will be half-way to ——'—naming the local mental hospital.

SITUATION AT FOLLOW-UP

Age: nine years
Average improvement/deterioration rating = 0 (the same)

CHANGES IN FAMILY BACKGROUND

The paternal grandfather, who was blind, and had had a stroke, now stayed alternately with this family and with another son. Mother found this a strain, as he had to sleep in the kitchen, would not get dressed during the day and complained of headaches if the children made a noise. She had gone out to work again during the follow-up period and had been in three different jobs within a twelve-month period. At the time she was not working, as her little boy had 'begun to suffer with his nerves', complaining of abdominal pains and refusing to leave the house after wetting his pants one day; he was still very worried about going on any outing where he might temporarily be out of reach of a lavatory. The mother, herself, was more relaxed and was no longer taking 'tranquillisers'.

PROGRESS OF ORIGINAL PROBLEMS

The child still suffered from asthma and eczema. The eczema appeared to be limited to her hands, between her fingers, but the mother was worried about it as, about twelve months previously, it had occurred in the same place and had turned into impetigo. The child still had asthmatic attacks but not perhaps so often as she had done previously. Recently, however, she

CLINIC CASE

plan of ignoring both asthma and eczema so far as was possible; for instance, the child was left to put ointment on the eczema herself.

Her general behaviour was still said to be 'very trying indeed'. The mother felt that 'she has got no sense' and, for instance, if she were out on her bicycle, the mother would worry all the time about the possibility of an accident. She did not worry in this way about any of the other children, but felt that this girl was the one 'who always does silly things'. She did not get on well with her siblings; she fought 'like cat and dog' with her older sister. She often wanted to go out with this sister and her friends, but they did not seem to want her and she usually finished up in tears, complaining that they were unkind to her. Similarly, her younger brother had his circle of friends, but they did not seem to encourage her to join it. She never appeared to have any friends of her own; she had told her mother that she did have friends at school, but they lived too far away to play with. She seemed to find it impossible to join in the other children's games but only to interfere with them. For instance, if they played cards, she would go round saying what was in other people's hands. She was said to have been very pleased about the arrival of the new baby. However, when she was allowed to hold him, 'she was not very kind to him'. On one occasion she had dropped him and on others she was believed to have smacked him because he cried.

She was very untruthful and would deny that she had done things and blame one of the other children with such conviction that sometimes the other child had been wrongly punished; she would swear that she had not done something, even under circumstances where confession would have brought much less trouble—for instance, if she had accidentally broken

MATCHED CHILD

had also tended to wake up in the morning wheezing and with running eyes and nose. This occurred in the winter as well as in the summer. There had not been any allergy tests done and the child slept on a flock mattress and shared a room with a sister who had feather pillows. The mother felt that the child was almost permanently 'wheezy' and frequently drew attention to this in front of her, e.g. by saying 'See how she breathes'.

She was still faddy about food, but on the whole seemed to be able to eat an average-size meal, though she did not have a big appetite. The mother was rather worried because 'she doesn't seem to grow at all' and, at the age of nine, was wearing clothes sized for a child two or three years younger. She talked with a faint lisp and in a rather babyish manner and, according to mother, still sucked her thumb fairly frequently. While sucking her thumb she still had to have a 'nose tickler', i.e. a bit of frayed woollen material, to hold crumpled in her hand at the same time. Without this she did not appear to get any satisfaction from the thumb-sucking.

She was inclined to be rather irritable at present, but this mainly took the form of mild crossness and she seldom had a real tantrum. She still argued a great deal with both her siblings, which continued to upset both parents and particularly father. She was easily upset by other people's unhappiness and would cry, for instance, if a person or animal was hurt on television. She had also cried recently because she was so sorry for her grandfather, who was blind and who had been staying with the family for three months. She was extremely afraid of the dark when she was in bed at night and had to have a light on in the hall, even though she slept in the same room as her older sister. If she woke during the night and found the light out she would call out to her father to put on his bedside lamp so

CLINIC CASE

a cup. She seemed to be always complaining that she was misused and seemed to think that the other children were receiving advantages denied to her. On the other hand, if she gained extra benefits, e.g. if she was first home from school and given the only sweet available, she would use this to provoke the other children by gloating over it in front of them. She had also caused embarassment to her parents by repeating things to relatives and neighbours. She was very destructive and when she had been given a toy typewriter for her birthday, had been found prising it apart with a metal ruler within a week. She was always losing her possessions, including clothes, and would then swear that someone else had stolen them or taken them from her. She cried a great deal, either through temper or because pressure was being put upon her to do something she did not wish to do.

Her school reports were, according to her mother, now showing her as being below average in attainment, but see the school report below. Mother had tried 'helping her' with reading at home, but this usually ended in a scene, as she did not concentrate but 'just looks round the room'.

SCHOOL REPORT

Attendance good; general attainment and reading ability average for her age; usually in the middle 50 per cent of her teaching group; very restless; sucks her thumb; very irritable; aggressive towards other children.

FAMILY ATTITUDE

The mother's attitude was now approaching open rejection. She complained of the child's behaviour and ailments as if they were being done out of deliberate malice towards herself. For instance, both the other girls in the family also had eczema, but mother said: 'I don't feel so bad about it with them.' She also had a great fear of

MATCHED CHILD

that she could then go and turn on the landing light for herself. She still had occasional nightmares. There had been no recurrence of her reluctance to go to school and she now appeared to like it very much.

SCHOOL REPORT

Attendance was good; attainment average for age; usually in the middle 50 per cent of her teaching group; she worried more than other children; 'she needs and seeks attention; is a help in class on many occasions'.

FAMILY ATTITUDE

Mother still showed a tendency to stress the child's defects even in her presence; her 'wheezing', her 'dry skin, like an old woman's', and her smallness were all mentioned. She was also said to be 'rather slow' at school, though there was no question of this from the school report. On the other hand, the child was also credited

CLINIC CASE	MATCHED CHILD
the child being hurt or killed if, for instance, she went out on her father's motor-cycle: a fear that did not occur in respect of any of the other children. She was making very strong efforts to avoid jealousy-provoking situations between her two youngest children, and now thought that this girl's problems were due to her failure to do this when the child was small.	with good points; for instance, she was said to be very helpful in the house. This mother said frankly that she never wanted children and there appeared to be mild generalised rejection of all three children rather than the open personal rejection of one child which was noted of the clinic case.

Appendix Three

Questionnaires

1. Administered to parents initially (page 212)
2. Administered to parents at follow-up (page 216)
3. Administered to teachers (page 220)

Serial No...............................

BUCKINGHAMSHIRE CHILD SURVEY

A

Below are some descriptions of illnesses and health problems which can affect children. If any item is true of your child, will you please put a line under **Yes.** If the item does not apply to your child then please put the line under **No.**

This child

1. Wears glasses always .... Yes No
2. Wears glasses sometimes .... Yes No
3. Is having treatment for eyes at clinic or hospital .... Yes No
4. Has had persistent ear-ache or running ear during the last twelve months .... Yes No
5. Seems to have difficulty in hearing sometimes Yes No
6. Has a hearing aid .... Yes No
7. Suffers from sick headaches .... Yes No
8. Gets travel sick in car, bus or train .... Yes No
9. Has frequent colds or sore throats .... Yes No
10. Has a persistent and troublesome cough .... Yes No
11. Is overweight .... Yes No
12. Is underweight .... Yes No
13. Has fainted more than twice in life .... Yes No
14. Is highly strung .... Yes No
15. Has suffered from a rash or other skin trouble which lasted for two weeks or longer .... Yes No
16. Has to wear special support for bone or muscle disorder (for instance, iron on leg, built up shoe, etc.) .... Yes No
17. Has to wear brace on teeth .... Yes No
18. Has a stammer .... Yes No

Has a **doctor** ever said that this child suffered from

19. Any disease or disorder of the bones (*Not* a broken bone) .... Yes No
20. Any disease or disorder affecting muscles .... Yes No
21. Heart trouble .... Yes No
22. Eczema .... Yes No
23. Asthma .... Yes No
24. Tuberculosis .... Yes No
25. Any chronic lung trouble (such as chronic Bronchitis) .... Yes No
26. St. Vitus Dance .... Yes No
27. Meningitis (Brain Fever) .... Yes No
28. Migraine .... Yes No
29. Cerebral Palsy ("Spastic") .... Yes No
30. Fits or Convulsions .... Yes No
31. Diabetes .... Yes No
32. Rheumatic Fever .... Yes No
33. Hare-lip or cleft palate .... Yes No
34. Any disorder of the glands (*not* just swollen neck glands) .... Yes No
35. Any other physical handicap or **chronic** illness Yes No
If so, what is it? Please write it below.

....

....

....

For Girls only:

36. Have periods started yet? .... Yes No
37. At what age was first period (write in number) ....
38. If periods have started, does she
(*a*) Worry about it.
(*b*) Feel sick.
(*c*) Complain of pains.
(*d*) Have to stay away from school or go to bed.
(*e*) Usually have no trouble or worry at all.

Please underline any of these items which you think apply to this girl

For Boys only:

39. Has his voice broken yet? .... Yes No
40. If so, at what age did this happen? ....
41. Has this child ever had any illness or operation which made it necessary to stay in hospital for more than one night? .... Yes No. If so, please fill in the details below.

	Age when went to hospital	*How long stayed there*	*Name of illness, accident or operation*
42.	....	....	....
	....	....	....
	....	....	....
	....	....	....

43. If the child has been in hospital, did you find that behaviour had changed in any way immediately after return home?

....

....

....

44. Has this child ever attended a special school or class because of a health problem (hearing, sight, speech, etc.)? If so, please tell us about it.

....

....

....

Open to next page

B

Below are some statements which describe the way that children behave. In each group of three, please underline the description that best suits your child at the present time.

45. Seldom or never purposely destroys things.
About as destructive as most children of the same age.
Very destructive.

46. Very much afraid of one or more animals (that is ordinary British animals, not lions, tigers, etc.).
A little afraid of some animals.
Not at all afraid of animals.

47. Has no fear of meeting new people.
A little afraid or shy of new people.
Generally fearful of unfamiliar people.

48. Afraid of the dark when in bed at night.
Seems a little uneasy unless a dim light is left on.
Has no fear of the dark.

49. Always tells the truth.
Tells an occasional fib.
Tells deliberate untruths quite often.

50. Likes school very much.
Likes school about as much as most children.
Dislikes going to school.

51. Never takes anything that belongs to someone else.
Has helped himself to someone else's things at least once or twice (including taking things belonging to other members of the family).
Has stolen things on several occasions.

52. Very irritable, easily becomes cross or annoyed.
Occasionally becomes cross (for instance, if tired or provoked by other children).
Very placid nature, practically never gets cross or annoyed.

53. Rather fussy about food, will eat only certain things.
Has fairly definite food preferences but will eat most foods if hungry.
Will eat nearly anything.

54. Not at all shy, mixes freely with other children.
A little shy with strange children.
Very shy, bashful, fearful of other children.

55. Always hungry, eats a great deal both at meals and as snacks between meals. Can't stop him eating.
Eats about as much as others of the same age.
Small appetite, inclined to pick at food.

56. Very carefree, doesn't worry about anything.
Occasionally worries (for instance, about tests at school or illness in the family).
Often seems worried, worries about many things.

57. Complains and whines a lot, hard to satisfy.
Complains about as much as most children of the same age.
Seldom or never complains or whines.

58. Very restless and fidgety, cannot sit still for a minute.
About as active as most children of the same age.
Less active than average, likes sitting still as much as possible.

59. Tends to be very jealous.
Occasionally shows jealousy.
Seldom or never jealous.

60. Never wanders off from home without saying where going.
Loiters on way home from school or may go to play with friends without telling parents.
Wanders off for long distances or long periods without parents knowing where.

61. Almost daily has times of being drawn into self and out of touch with other people.
Occasionally seems lost in a dream world.
Seldom or never day dreams.

62. Always does things when told.
About as obedient as most children.
Usually resists when asked or told to do things.

63. Plays truant from school more than once or twice a month.
Plays truant more than three to four times a year.
Never plays truant.

Go to next page

Below is a list of minor health problems which most children have at some time. Please tell us how often each of these happens to your child by putting a tick (√) in the appropriate column.

Example. If your child complains of headaches about once a month you would put the tick (√) in column (*e*) where it says "About once a month". If your child has only had a headache once or twice in his or her whole life, then you would put the tick (√) in column (*h*) where it says "Never or less than once a year".

	(*a*) *Every day or almost every day,*	(*b*) *Two or three times a week.*	(*c*) *About once a week.*	(*d*) *About once every two weeks.*	(*e*) *About once a month.*	(*f*) *About once in two or three months.*	(*g*) *Two or three times a year.*	(*h*) *Never, or less than once a year.*
68. Has constipation								
69. Has headaches								
70. Has nightmares or unpleasant or frightening dreams								
71. Is restless in sleep, tosses and turns, kicks off bedclothes, or walks in sleep, etc. ...								
72. Wets the bed								
73. Has pains in stomach								
74. Vomits								
75. Has diarrhea								
76. Poor control of bowels, soils self								
77. Cries								
78. Sulks for hours on end								
79. Has real temper tantrums (that is complete loss of temper with shouting, angry movements, etc.)								
80. Bites nails								
81. Sucks thumb or finger								
82. Has bitter quarrels with other children ...								

Turn to next page

64. Has a very noticeable twitch of face or body, or mannerism, which takes place most of the time.
Has occasional twitches or mannerisms which occur when tired, bored, etc.
Has no twitches or mannerisms.

65. Moods very changeable, on top of the world one minute, down the next for no particular reason.
Occasional changes of mood in response to things that happen.
Runs on very even keel, always the same except under very unusual circumstances.

66. Seemed to have difficulty in learning to read.
Learned to read as quickly as most children.
Good reader, learned to read more quickly than other children.

67. Is there anything about your child's behaviour or habits which worries you but which we have not mentioned?
If so, please tell us about it here..

....

....

....

C

Thank you for telling us about your child. Now, to finish, could you please give us some information about the child's background as this will help us a great deal when we come to compare the answers of all our parents.

83. What was this child's age **last** birthday? ....

84. Is this child a boy or a girl? ....

85. Is the person answering these questions the child's mother?..............................Yes No
If not, please explain who it is.

....

86. How many **other** children are there in the family? ....Boys
..............................Girls.

87. Is the child's father alive? .... If so, what is his age? ....

88. Is the child's mother alive? .... If so, what is her age? ....

89. Is this child
(*a*) The only one.
(*b*) The youngest.
(*c*) The oldest.
(*d*) In the middle.

Please underline the description that applies.

90. What is the name of your husband's job?..
Please describe what he does..

....

....

91. Besides being a mother, do **you** have a job?
(*a*) Full-time?
(*b*) Part-time?
(*c*) Not at all?

92. How long have you lived in the district in which you live now?

....

93. Where did you live before that? *(Just give the name of the town or village* not *your address)*

....

94. Has either parent been away from home (for instance, in hospital) for more than a month since this child's birth? Yes No
If so, was it Father/Mother? (*Please underline right word.*)

95. Apart from any visits to hospital (which you have already described) has the child lived away from home (for instance, with relatives) for more than a month at at any one time? If so, please tell us about it.

....

....

....

....

THANK YOU VERY MUCH.

PLEASE DO NOT SIGN YOUR NAME.

Serial No...

BUCKINGHAMSHIRE CHILD SURVEY

A

Below are some descriptions of illnesses and health problems which can affect children. If any item is true of your child, will you please put a line under **Yes.** If the item does not apply to your child then please put the line under **No.**

This child

1. Seems to have difficulty in hearing sometimes Yes No
2. Suffers from sick headaches .... Yes No
3. Gets travel sick in car, bus, or train .... Yes No
4. Has frequent colds or sore throats .... Yes No
5. Has a persistent and troublesome cough.............. Yes No
6. Is overweight .... Yes No
7. Is underweight .... Yes No
8. Is highly strung .... Yes No
9. Has a stammer.............................. Yes No
10. Has had eczema during the last year .... Yes No
11. Has had asthma during the last year .... Yes No
12. Has any physical handicap or chronic illness Yes No
    If so, what is it? Please write it below

....

....

....

For Girls only:

13. Have periods started yet?..............................Yes No
14. At what age was first period (write in number)..............................
15. If periods have started does she
    (*a*) Worry about it.
    (*b*) Feel sick.
    (*c*) Complain of pain.
    (*d*) Have to stay away from school or go to bed.
    (*e*) Usually have no trouble or worry at all.

Please underline any of these items which you think apply to this girl.

16. **During the last three years,** has this child had any illness or operation which made it necessary to stay in hospital for more than one night?..............................Yes No. If so, please fill in the details below.

Age when went to hospital	*How long stayed there*	*Name of illness, accident or operation*
....	....	....
....	....	....
....	....	....

17. During the last three years, has this child been seen by a specialist doctor as an outpatient at a hospital or clinic?

Type of clinic	*What was the problem?*	*Dates attended (approx.)* *From*	*To*
....	....	....	
....	....	....	
....	....	....	
....	....	....	

18. During the last three years, has this child been treated by his Family Doctor for any serious illness or persistent problem? If so, please tell us about it.

....

....

....

19. During the last three years, has this child attended any special school or class because of a health problem (hearing, speech, etc.)?..............................Yes No. If so, what was it?

....

....

....

20. During the last three years, has any **other** member of the household been in hospital or had any **serious** illness at home?
..............................Yes No. If so, please give details below.

Relationship to child (e.g. Grandmother, Brother)	*Date (Year)*	*Name of illness*	*How long ill?*	*In hospital how long?*
....	....	....	....	....
....	....	....	....	....
....	....	....	....	....
....	....	....	....	....

Open to next page

B

Below are some statements which describe the way that children behave. In each group of three, please underline the description that best suits <u>your</u> child at the present time.

21. Seldom or never purposely destroys things.
About as destructive as most children of the same age.
Very destructive.

22. Very much afraid of one or more animals (that is ordinary British animals, not lions, tigers, etc.).
A little afraid of some animals.
Not at all afraid of animals.

23. Has no fear of meeting new people.
A little afraid or shy of new people.
Generally fearful of unfamiliar people.

24. Afraid of the dark when in bed at night.
Seems a little uneasy unless a dim light is left on.
Has no fear of the dark.

25. Always tells the truth.
Tells an occasional fib.
Tells deliberate untruths quite often.

26. Likes school very much.
Likes school about as much as most children.
Dislikes going to school.

27. Never takes anything that belongs to someone else.
Has helped himself to someone else's things at least once or twice (including taking things belonging to other members of the family).
Has stolen things on several occasions.

28. Very irritable, easily becomes cross or annoyed.
Occasionally becomes cross (for instance, if tired or provoked by other children).
Very placid nature, practically never gets cross or annoyed.

29. Rather fussy about food, will eat only certain things.
Has fairly definite food preferences but will eat most foods if hungry.
Will eat nearly anything.

30. Not at all shy, mixes freely with other children.
A little shy with strange children.
Very shy, bashful, fearful of other children.

31. Always hungry, eats a great deal both at meals and as snacks between meals. Can't stop him eating.
Eats about as much as others of the same age.
Small appetite, inclined to pick at food.

32. Very carefree, doesn't worry about anything.
Occasionally worries (for instance, about tests at school or illness in the family).
Often seems worried, worries about many things.

33. Complains and whines a lot, hard to satisfy.
Complains about as much as most children of the same age.
Seldom or never complains or whines.

34. Very restless and fidgety, cannot sit still for a minute.
About as active as most children of the same age.
Less active than average, likes sitting still as much as possible

35. Tends to be very jealous.
Occasionally shows jealousy.
Seldom or never jealous.

36. Never wanders off from home without saying where going.
Loiters on way home from school or may go to play with friends without telling parents.
Wanders off for long distances or long periods without parents knowing where.

37. Almost daily has times of being drawn into self and out of touch with other people.
Occasionally seems lost in a dream world.
Seldom or never day dreams.

38. Always does things when told.
About as obedient as most children.
Usually resists when asked or told to do things.

39. Plays truant from school more than once or twice a month.
Plays truant more than three to four times a year.
Never plays truant.

Go to next page

Below is a list of minor health problems which most children have at some time. Please tell us how often each of these happens to this child by putting a tick (√) in the appropriate column.

Example. If this child complains of headaches about once a month you would put the tick (√) in column (*e*) where it says "About once a month". If this child has only had a headache once or twice in his or her whole life, then you would put the tick (√) in column (*h*) where it says "Never or less than once a year".

	(*a*) *Every day or almost every day.*	(*b*) *Two or three times a week.*	(*c*) *About once a week.*	(*d*) *About once every two weeks.*	(*e*) *About once a month.*	(*f*) *About once in two or three months.*	(*g*) *Two or three times a year.*	(*h*) *Never, or less than once a year.*
40. Has constipation								
41. Has headaches								
42. Has nightmares or unpleasant or frightening dreams								
43. Is restless in sleep, tosses and turns, kicks off bedclothes, or walks in sleep, etc. ...								
44. Wets the bed								
45. Has pains in stomach								
46. Vomits								
47. Has diarrhoea								
48. Poor control of bowels, soils self								
49. Cries								
50. Sulks for hours on end								
51. Has real temper tantrums (that is complete loss of temper with shouting, angry movements, etc.)								
52. Bites nails								
53. Sucks thumb or finger								
54. Has bitter quarrels with other children ...								

Go to next page

55. Has a very noticeable twitch of face or body, or mannerism, which takes place most of the time.
Has occasional twitches or mannerisms which occur when tired, bored, etc.
Has no twitches or mannerisms.

56. Moods very changeable, on top of the world one minute, down the next for no particular reason.
Occasional changes of mood in response to things that happen.
Runs on very even keel, always the same except under very unusual circumstances.

57. Seemed to have difficulty in learning to read.
Learned to read as quickly as most children.
Good reader, learned to read more quickly than other children.

58. Is there anything about your child's behaviour or habits which worries you but which we have not mentioned?
If so, please tell us about it here..........

....

....

....

C

Thank you for telling us about your child. Now, to finish, could you please give us some information about the child's background as this will help us a great deal when we come to compare the answers of all our parents.

59. What was this child's age **last** birthday? ....

60. Is the person answering these questions the child's mother?..........Yes No
If not, please explain who it is.

....

61. How many **other** children are there in the family?..........Boys. Ages..........
..........Girls. Ages..........

62. Is the child's father alive?.......... If he is dead or has left home permanently, when did this happen?
Died.......... Left home..........

63. Is the child's mother alive?.......... If she is dead or has left home permanently, when did this happen?
Died.......... Left home..........

64. During the last three years, has any other member of the household died?..........Yes No. Has any other friend or relative died who did not live with you but of whom the child was very fond?..........Yes No. Please tell us who died and when?

....

....

....

65. What is the name of your husband's job?..........
Please describe what he does..........

....

....

66. Besides being a mother, do **you** have a job?
(*a*) Full-time?
(*b*) Part-time?
(*c*) Not at all?

67. During the last three years, has the child spent any time longer than a week away from home (apart from stays in hospital which you have already described)?..........Yes No. If so, please tell us about it.

Age when went away	*Reason* (e.g. holiday, mother's illness, etc.)	*With whom did he/she stay?* (e.g. Aunt, Children's Home, etc.)	*How long was he/she away?*
....	....	....	....
....	....	....	....
....	....	....	....

68. Has either parent been away from home (apart from hospital) for a month or more during the last three years? Yes/No..........
If so, was it Father/Mother? *(Please underline right word.)*

THANK YOU VERY MUCH.

PLEASE DO NOT SIGN YOUR NAME.

CONFIDENTIAL *Serial No.................*

BUCKINGHAMSHIRE CHILD SURVEY

Name of child ....

Address ....

School ....Class ....

A. Attendance

1. Number of attendances credited during last *complete* term ....

2. Total number of possible attendances during that term ....

3. *Please underline* any of the following reasons for absence which you believe apply to this child:
   - (a) Genuine illness of child
   - (b) Illness of parent or other member of family
   - (c) Parental holiday taken during school term
   - (d) Periodic visits to hospital, clinic, etc.
   - (e) Truanting (absence without parental permission)
   - (f) Odd days and half days off for no good reason but apparently with support and knowledge of parents
   - (g) Any other reason (please specify) ....

   ....

B. Attainment

1. Age range in child's class .... 2. Child's age ....

3. Is this child's place in class or teaching group usually in (a) Top 25%
   (*please underline*) (b) Middle 50%
   (c) Bottom 25%

4. If there is more than one stream for this age group, is streaming
   - (a) Parallel
   - (b) Based on merit (*please underline*)
   - (c) Based on month of birth?

   If merit streaming is used, how does this child's class compare with others in the same year

   (e.g. middle of three, second of five, etc.) ....

   ....

5. *Please underline* in each question below the item which best fits this child:
   - (a) General attainment level above average for age, and type of school
     General attainment level average for age, and type of school
     General attainment level below average for age, and type of school
   - (b) Has not yet learned to read
     Reading ability below average for age
     Reading ability average for age
     Reading ability above average for age

6. Has this child been given any intelligence or other standardized tests (for instance of reading age) at school? If so, please give details below.

Name of Test	*Child's Age at Test*	*Result (IQ, Reading Age, etc.)*
....	....	....
....	....	....
....	....	....

P.T.O.

C. Behaviour and Health Problems

1. *Please underline*, in the list below, any items which describe this child as he often is:

(a) Very restless, can't sit still for a moment
(b) Cries more than most children
(c) Has a stammer
(d) Has other speech difficulty
(e) Often tells lies
(f) Has stolen things on one or more occasions
(g) Is very easily frightened
(h) Bites finger nails
(i) Sucks thumb or finger
(j) Very irritable, easily becomes cross or annoyed
(k) Has had one or more temper tantrums at school during this year
(l) Is unco-operative in class
(m) Very shy, finds it difficult to mix with other children
(n) Has wet or soiled self at school during last year
(o) Has noticeable twitch of face or body
(p) Worries more than other children
(q) Aggressive towards other children
(r) Very quiet or withdrawn
(s) Very moody—on top of world one minute, down the next
(t) Not interested in school work
(u) Has on one or more occasions during this school year shown fear of school—that is, tears on arrival or refusal to come into the building.

2. Has this child, to the best of your knowledge, any medical disability or chronic illness? (Please do *not* ask the child.) If so, what is it? Does it affect performance or participation in school activities?

....

....

....

D. Other Comments

If there is any other information about this child which we have not covered but which you feel to be relevant (e.g. home conditions), please use this space to tell us about it.

....

....

....

....

....

....

....

....

....

....

Bibliography

ACKERSON, L. (1931) *Children's behaviour problems I: Incidence, genetic and intellectual factors*. Chicago: Chicago University Press.

ACKERSON, L. (1942) *Children's behaviour problems II: Relative importance and interrelations among traits*. Chicago: Chicago University Press.

ADDIS, R. S. (1935) 'A statistical study of nocturnal enuresis.' *Arch. Dis. Child.*, **10**, 169.

ARIES, P. (1965) *Centuries of childhood: a social history of family life*. New York: Vintage Books.

BAIN, W. E. (1934) 'A study of attitude of teachers toward behaviour problems.' *Child Develop.*, **5**, 19.

BAKWIN, H., and BAKWIN, R. M. (1954) *Behaviour disorders in childhood*. London: Saunders.

BALDWIN, A. L. (1944) 'An analysis of children's eating habits.' *J. Pediat.*, **25**, 74.

BALDWIN, A. L., KALHORN, J., and BRESSE, F. H. (1945) *Patterns of parent behaviour*. Evanston, Illinois: American Psychological Association.

BALDWIN, A. L. (1947) 'Changes in parent behaviour during pregnancy: an experiment in longitudinal analysis.' *Child Develop.*, **18**, 29.

BARBOUR, R. F. (1951) in Child Guidance Inter-Clinic Conference, *9th. Follow-up on child guidance cases*. London: National Association for Mental Health.

BARBOUR, R. F., and BEEDELL, C. J. (1955) 'The follow-up of a child guidance clinic population.' *J. ment. Sci.*, **101**, 794.

BARBOUR, R. F., BORLAND, E. M., BOYD, M. M., MILLER, A., and OPPE, T. T. (1963) 'Enuresis as a disorder of development.' *Brit. med. J.*, **2**, 437.

BELL, R. Q. (1959–60) 'Retrospective and prospective views of early personality development.' *Merrill-Palmer Q. Behav. & Develop.*, **6**, 131.

BILLIG, A. L. (1941) 'Finger nail-biting: its incipiency, incidence and amelioration.' *Genet. Psychol. Monogr.*, **24**, 123.

BIRCH, L. B. (1955) 'The incidence of nail-biting among school children.' *Brit. J. educ. Psychol.*, **25**, 123.

BLATZ, W. E., and BOTT, E. A. (1927) 'Studies in mental hygiene: I Behaviour of public school children.' *Ped. Sem. & J. genet. Psychol.*, **34**, 552.

BLOMFIELD, J. M., and DOUGLAS, J. W. B. (1956) 'Bed-wetting: Prevalence among children aged 4–7 years.' *Lancet*, **1**, 856.

BOWER, E. M. (1958) 'A process for early identification of emotionally disturbed children.' *Bull. Calif. State Dept. Educ.*, **27**, 6.

BOWER, E. M. (1961) 'Primary prevention in a school setting.' In CAPLAN, G. (ed.) *Prevention of mental disorder in children*. London: Tavistock Publications.

BOWER, E. M. (1962) 'Comparison of the characteristics of identified emotionally disturbed children with other children in classes.' In TRAPP, E. P., and HIMELSTEIN, P. (eds.) *Readings on the exceptional child*. London: Methuen.

BRANDON, S. (1960) 'An epidemiological study of maladjustment in childhood.' M. D. Thesis. University of Durham (King's College Newcastle.)

BRANSBY, E. R., BLOMFIELD, J. M., and DOUGLAS, J. W. B. (1955) 'The prevalence of bed-wetting.' *Med. Offr.*, **44**, 5.

BREMER, J. (1951) 'A social psychiatric investigation of a small community in Northern Norway.' *Acta Psychiat. Neurol. Suppl.*, 62.

BUCKLE, D., and LEBOVICI, S. (1960) *Child guidance centres*. Geneva: World Health Organization.

BURT, C. (1917) *The distribution and relations of educational abilities*. London: London County Council.

BURT, C. (1935) *The subnormal mind*. London: Oxford University Press.

CATTELL, R. B., and COAN, R. W. (1957) 'Personality factors in middle childhood as revealed in parents ratings.' *Child Develop.*, **28**, 4.

CHAZAN, M. (1962) 'School phobia.' *Brit. J. educ. Psychol.*, **32**, 209.

CHAZAN, M. (1963) 'Maladjustment, attainment and sociometric status.' Univ. Coll. Swansea. *Faculty of Education Journal*, **4**, 7.

CHAZAN, M. (1968) 'Children's emotional development.' In BUTCHER, H. J. (ed.) *Educational Research in Britain*. London: University of London Press Ltd.

CHESS, S., THOMAS, A., and BIRCH, H. G. (1959) 'Characteristics of the individual child's behavioural responses to the environment.' *Amer. J. Orthopsychiat.*, **29**, 791.

CHESS, S., THOMAS, A., RUTTER, M., and BIRCH, H. G. (1963) 'Interaction of temperament and environment in the production of behavioural disturbance in children.' *Amer. J. Psychiat.*, **120**, 142.

CHESS, S., THOMAS, A., and BIRCH, H. G. (1967) 'Behaviour problems revisited: Findings of an anterospective study.' *J. Amer. Acad. Child Psychiat.*, **6**, 321.

COHEN, H. (1955) 'The evolution of the concept of disease.' *Proc. Roy. Soc. Med.*, **48**, 155.

COOLIDGE, J. C., BRODIE, R. D., and FEENEY, B. (1964) 'A ten-year follow-up of sixty-six school-phobic children.' *Amer. J. Orthopstchiat.*, **4**, 675.

CRANDALL, V. J., and PRESTON, A. (1955) 'Patterns and levels of maternal behaviour.' *Child Develop.*, **26**, 267.

CUMMINGS, J. D. (1944) 'Emotional symptoms in school children.' *Brit. J. educ. Psychol.*, **14**, 151.

CUMMINGS, J. D. (1946) 'A follow-up study of emotional symptoms in schoolchildren.' *Brit. J. educ. Psychol.*, **16**, 163.

CUNNINGHAM, J. M., WESTERMAN, H. H., and FISCHHOFF, J. (1956) 'A follow-up study of patients seen in a psychiatric clinic for children.' *Amer. J. Orthopsychiat.* **26**, 602.

CYTRYN, L., GILBERT, A., and EISENBERG, L. (1960) 'The effectiveness of tranquilizing drugs plus supportive psychotherapy in testing behaviour disorders of children.' *Amer. J. Orthopsychiat.*, **30**, 113.

DAVIDSON, M. (1961) 'Einige Untersuchungsergebnisse über psychologische Störungen bei Kindern.' *Praxis der Kinderpsychologie*, **10**, 273.

DEL SOLAR, C. (1949) *Parents and teachers view the child: a comparative study of parents' and teachers' appraisals of children.* Bureau of Publications, Teachers College, Columbia University.

DOUGLAS, J. W. B., and MULLIGAN, D. G. (1961) 'Emotional adjustment and educational achievement—the preliminary results of a longitudinal study of a national sample of children.' *Proc. Roy. Soc. Med.*, 54, 885.

DOUGLAS, J. W. B. (1964) *The home and the school.* London: MacGibbon and Kee.

EISENBERG, L. (1958) 'School phobia: A study in the communication of anxiety.' *Amer. J. Psychiat.*, **114**, 712.

EISENBERG, L. (1961) 'The effectiveness of psychotherapy alone and in lone conjunction with perphenazine or placebo in the treatment of neurotic and hyperkimatic children.' *Amer. J. Psychiat.*, **117**, 1088.

ELLIS, D. B., and MILLER, L. W. (1936) 'Teachers' attitudes and child behaviour problems.' *J. educ. Psychol.*, **27**, 501.

ERON, L. D., WALDER, L. O., LAULIGHT, J. H., and HLADKY, F. (1958) 'The psychosocial development of aggressive behaviour in children.' *Proc. Rip Van Winkle Clinic*, **9**. 10.

ESTES, H. R., HAYLETT, C. H., and JOHNSON, A. M. (1956) 'Separation anxiety.' *Amer. J. Psychother.*, **10**, 682.

EYSENCK, H. J. (1952) 'The effects of psychotherapy: an evaluation.' *J. Consult. Psychol.* **16**, 319.

EYSENCK, H. J. (1953) *The structure of human personality*. London: Methuen.

EYSENCK, H. J., and COOKSON, D. (1969) 'Personality in primary school children: 2 Teachers' ratings.' *Brit. J. educ. Psychol.*, **39**, 123.

FITT, A. B. (1956) 'An experimental study of children's attitude to school in Auckland, New Zealand.' *Brit. J. educ. Psychol.*, **26**, 25.

FOSTER, J. C., and ANDERSON, J. E. (1930) *The young child and his parents: a study of one hundred cases.* (Institute of Child Welfare, Monograph Series, Number 1) University of Minnesota.

FRICK, W. B. (1964) 'School phobia: a critical review of the literature.' *Merrill-Palmer Q. Behav. & Develop.*, **10**, 361.

FURMAN, S. S., SWEAT, L. G., and CROCETTI, G. M. (1965) 'Social class factors in the flow of children to outpatient psychiatric facilities.' *Amer. J. Public Health*, **55**, 385.

GARDNER, G. (1953) *Psychiatric treatment.* New York: Williams and Williams.

GEDDA, E. (1948) 'De cas notés de troubles de canduite nerveux chez des élèves dans la periode commencants d'un district scoliare de Göteborg.' *Acta Paediat.*, **35**, 49.

GESELL, A. (1925) *The mental growth of the pre-school child.* London: MacMillan.

GESELL, A. (1940) *The first five years of life*. London: Methuen.

GESELL, A. (1956) *Youth: The years from ten to sixteen*. London: Methuen.

GESELL, A., and ILG, F. L. (1946) *The child from five to ten*. London: Methuen.

GILBERT, G. M. (1957) 'A survey of "referral problems" in metropolitan child guidance centres.' *J. clin. Psychol.*, **13**, 37.

GLASER, K. (1959) 'Problems in school attendance: school phobia and related conditions.' *Pediatrics*, **23**, 371.

GLIDEWELL, J. C., MENSH, I. N., and GILDEA, M. C. -L. (1957) 'Behaviour symptoms in children and degree of sickness.' *Amer. J. Psychiat.*, **114**, 47.

GLIDEWELL, J. C., GILDEA, M. C. -L., DOMKE, H. R., and KANTOR, M. B. (1960) 'Behaviour symptoms in children and adjustment in public school.' *Human Organization*, **18**, 123.

GLIDEWELL, J. C., DOMKE, H. R., and KANTOR, M. B. (1963) 'Screening in schools for behaviour disorders: use of mothers' reports of symptoms.' *J. educ. Res.*, **56**, 508.

GLIDEWELL, J. C. (1966) 'Studies of mothers' reports of behaviour symptoms in their children.' (Unpublished report).

GOLDBERG, D. P. (1969) 'The identification and assessment on non-psychotic illness by means of a questionnaire.' D. M. Thesis, University of Oxford.

GOLDFARB, A. (1963) 'Teacher ratings in psychiatric case-findings: I Methodical considerations.' *Amer. J. Public Health*, **53**, 1919.

GOODENOUGH, F. (1931) *Anger in young children*. Minneapolis: University of Minnesota Press.

GORDON, I. (1942) 'Allergy, enuresis and stammering.' *Brit. med. J.*, **1**, 357.

GORDON, J. E. (1957) 'The validity of Shoben's parent attitude survey.' *J. clin. Psychol.*, **13**, 154.

GRANT, Q. A. F. R. (1958) 'Age, and sex trends in the symptomatology of disturbed children.' Dissertation for the University of London Diploma of Psychological Medicine.

GRIFFITHS, W. (1952) *Behaviour difficulties of children as perceived and judged by parents, teachers and children themselves*. Minneapolis: University of Minnesota Press.

GUTTMAN, L. (1950) 'The basis for scalogram analysis.' In STOUFFAR, S. A. (ed.) *Measurement and prediction*. Princeton, N. J.: Princeton University Press.

HAGGERTY, M. E. (1925) 'The lucidence of undesirable behaviour in public school children.' *J. educ. Res.*, **12**, 102.

HALL, J., and JONES, D. C. (1950) 'Social grading of occupations.' *Brit. J. Sociol.*, **1**, 31.

HALLGREN, B. (1956) 'Enuresis. I A study with reference to the morbidity risk and symptomatology.' *Acta psychiat. et neurol.*, **31**, 379.

HEALD, F. B., MASLAND, R. P., STURGIS, S. H., and GALLAGHER, G. H. (1957) 'Dysmenorrhoea in adolescence.' *Pediatrics*, **20**, 121.

HERSOV, L. A. (1961a) 'Persistent non-attendance at school.' *J. Child Psychol.* Psychiat., **1**, 130.

HERSOV, I. A. (1961b) 'Refusal to go to school.' *J. Child Psychol. Psychiat.*, **1**, 137.

HEWITT, L. E., and JENKINS, R. L. (1946) *Fundamental patterns of maladjustment: the dynamics of their origin.* State of Illinois, Michigan Child Guidance Institute.

HILDRETH, G. (1928) 'A survey of problem pupils.' *J. educ. Res.*, **18**, 1.

HINDLEY, C. B. (1965) 'Stability and change in abilities up to five years: group trends.' *J. Child Psychol. Psychiat.*, **6**, 85.

HINDLEY, C. B. (1968) 'Growing up in five countries: a comparison of data on weaning, elimination training, age of walking and I.Q. in relation to social class from European longitudinal studies.' *Develop. Med. Child Neurol.*, **10**, 715.

HUBBARD, R. M., and ADAMS, C. F. (1936) 'Factors effecting success of child guidance clinic treatment.' *Amer. J. Orthopsychiat.*, **6**, 81.

HUNT, W. A., WITTSON, C. L., and HUNT, E. B. (1955) 'The relationship between amount of presenting symptomatology and severity of disability.' *J. clin. Psychol.*, **11**, 305.

HUNTER, E. C. (1957) 'Changes in teachers' attitudes toward children's behaviour over the last 30 years.' *Ment. Hyg.*, **41**, 3.

ILLINGWORTH, R. S. (1958) 'Obesity.' *J. Pediat.*, **53**, 117.

ISAACS, S. (1933) *Social development in young children.* London: Routledge, and Kegan Paul.

JERSILD, A. T., and HOLMES, F. B. (1935) 'Children's fears.' *Child Develop. Monogr.*, no. 20.

KANE, R. P., and CHAMBERS, G. S. (1961) 'Improvement—real or apparent.' *Amer. J. Psychiat.*, **117**, 1023.

KANNER, L. (1957) *Child psychiatry.* (Third edition). Oxford: Blackwell Scientific Publications.

KANNER, L. (1960) 'Do behavioural symptoms always indicate psychopathology?' *Child Psychol. & Psychiat.*, **1**, 17.

KANNER, L. (1962) 'Emotionally disturbed children: a historical review.' *Child Develop.*, **33**, 97.

KEIR, G. (1952) 'A history of child guidance.' *Brit. J. educ. Psychol.*, **22**, 5.

LAPOUSE, R., and MONK, M. (1958) 'An epidemiologic study of behaviour characteristics in children.' *Amer. J. Public Health*, **48**, 1134.

LAPOUSE, R., and MONK, M. (1959) 'Fears and worries in a representative sample of children.' *Amer. J. Orthopsychiat.*, **29**, 808.

LAPOUSE, R., and MONK, M. (1964) 'Behaviour deviations in a representative sample of children: variation by sex, age, race, social class and family size. *Amer. J. Orthopsychiat.*, **34**, 436.

LAPOUSE, R. (1965) 'The relationship of behaviour to adjustment in a representative sample of children.' *Amer. J. Public Health*, **55**, 1130.

LAYCOCK, S. R. (1934) 'Teachers' reactions to maladjustments of school children.' *Brit. J. educ. Psychol.*, **4**, 11.

LEVITT, E. E. (1957) 'The results of psychotherapy with children.' *J. Consult. Psychol.*, **21**, 189.

LEVY, D. M., and TULCHIN, S. H. (1932) 'The resistance of infants and children during mental health tests.' *J. exp. Psychol.*, **6**, 304.

LEVY, M. (1947) *Maternal over-protection.* New York: Columbia University Press.

LONG, A. (1941) 'Parents' reports of undesirable behaviour in children.' *Child Develop.*, **12**, 43.

LURIE, O. R. (1969) 'Emotional health of children in the family setting.' Paper presented at the Second International Congress of Social Psychiatry. (Unpublished).

MCCLURE, W. E. (1929) 'Characteristics of problem children based on judgements of teachers.' *J. juvenile Res.*, **13**, 124.

MCCONACHIE, J. W. (1955) In Ministry of Education. *Health of the school child.* London: HMSO.

MacFARLANE, J. W., ALLEN, L., and HONZIK, M. P. (1954) *A developmental study of the behaviour problems of normal children between 21 months and 14 years.* Berkeley and Los Angeles: University of California Press.

MCFIE, B. S. (1934) 'Behaviour and personality difficulties in school children.' *Brit. J. educ. Psychol.*, **4**, 30.

MACKENZIE, E. P. (1953) 'The treatment of anorexia.' *J. Pediat.*, **58**, 187.

MAES, W. R. (1966) 'The identification of emotionally disturbed elementary school children.' *Exceptional Children*, **32**, 607.

MALONE, A. J., and MASSLER, M. (1952) 'Index of nail-biting in children.' *J. abnorm. soc. Psychol.*, **47**, 193.

MANGUS, A. R. (1949) 'Mental health of rural children in Ohio.' *Res. Bull. Ohio Agricult. Exper. Sta.*, Research Bulletin 682.

MECHANIC, D. (1964) 'The influence of mothers on their children's health attitudes and behaviour.' *Pediatrics*, **33**, 444.

MEDICAL RESEARCH COUNCIL, Committee on Research into Chronic Bronchitis (1966) *Instructions for the use of the questionnaire on respiratory symptoms.* Medical Research Council.

MENSH, I. N., KANTOR, M. E., and DOMKE, H. R. (1959) 'Children's behaviour symptoms and their relationships to school adjustment, sex and social class.' *J. soc. Issues*, **15**, 8.

MICHAELS, J. J., and GOODMAN, S. E. (1934) 'Incidence and intercorrelations of enuresis and other neuropathic traits in so-called normal children.' *Amer. J. Orthopsychiat.*, **4**, 79.

MILLER, F. J. W., COURT, S. D. M., WALTON, W, S., and KNOX, E. G. (1960) *Growing up in Newcastle upon Tyne.* London: Oxford University Press.

Ministry of Education (1953) *Health of the school child, 1952–53.* Report of the Chief School Medical Officer for 1952–53. London: HMSO.

Ministry of Education (1955) *Report of the Committee on Maladjusted children.* (Underwood Report) London: HMSO.

MITCHELL, J. A. (1942) 'A study of teachers' and mental hygienists' ratings of certain behaviour problems of children.' *J. educ. Res.*, **36**, 292.

MITCHELL, S., and SHEPHERD, M. (1966) 'A comparative study of children's behaviour at home and at school.' *Brit. J. educ. Psychol.*, **36**, 248.

MITCHELL, S., and SHEPHERD, M. (1967) 'The child who dislikes going to school.' *Brit. J. educ. Psychol.*, **37**, 32.

MOORE, T., HINDLEY, C. B., and FALKNER, F. (1954) 'A longitudinal research in child development and some of its problems.' *Brit. med. J.*, **2**, 1132.

MOORE, T. W. (1959) 'Studying the growth of personality.' *Vita hum.*, 2, 65.

MOORE, T. W. (1965) 'The place of longitudinal research in the study of child development.' In MILLER, E. (ed.) *Foundations of child psychiatry.* Oxford: Pergamon Press.

MOORE, T. W. (1966) 'Difficulties of the ordinary child in adjusting to primary school.' *J. Child Psychol. Psychiat.*, **7**, 299.

MORRIS, D. P., SOROKER, E., and BURRUSS, G. (1954) 'Follow-up studies of shy withdrawn children—I Evaluation of later adjustment.' *Amer. J. Orthopsychiat.*, **24**, 743.

MORRIS, H. H., ESCOLI, P. J., and WEXLER, R. (1956) 'Aggressive behaviour disorders in childhood: a follow-up study.' *Amer. J. Psychiat.*, **112**, 991.

MORRIS, J. N. (1957) *Uses of epidemiology.* Livingstone: Edinburgh.

MULLEN, F. A. (1950) 'Truancy and classroom disorder as symptoms of personality problems.' *J. educ. Psychol.*, **41**, 97.

New York State Department of Mental Hygiene, Mental Health Research Unit (1964) 'Persistence of emotional disturbance reported among second and fourth grade children.' Onandage County School Studies, Interim report no. 1. (Mimeographed report).

NEWSON, J., and NEWSON, E. (1963) *Infant care in an urban community.* London: Allen & Unwin.

NEWSON, J., and NEWSON, E. (1968) *Four years old in an urban community.* London: Allen & Unwin.

NORRIS, V. (1951) 'Health of the schoolchild.' *Brit. J. soc. Med.*, **5**, 145.

OLSON, W. C. (1929) *Measurement of nervous habits in normal children.* University of Minneapolis Press.

OLSON, W. C. (1930) *Problem tendencies in children: a method for measurement and description.* University of Minneapolis Press.

O'NEAL, P., and ROBINS, L. N. (1958a) 'Childhood patterns predictive of adult schizophrenia: a 30-year follow-up study.' *Amer. J. Psychiat.*, **115**, 385.

O'NEAL, P., and ROBINS, L. N. (1958b) 'The relationship of childhood behaviour problems to adult psychiatric status: a 30-year follow-up study of 150 subjects.' *Amer. J. Psychiat.*, **114**, 961.

OPLER, M. K. (1969) 'Culture and child rearing.' In HOWELLS, J. G. (ed.) *Modern perspective in international child psychiatry.* Edinburgh: Oliver & Boyd.

PASAMANICK, B., and KAWI, A. (1956) 'A study of the association of prenatal and paranatal factors with the development of tics in children.' *J. Pediat.*, **48**, 596.

PETERSON, D. R., BECKER, W. C., SHOEMAKER, D. J., LURIA, Z., and HELLMER, L. A. (1961) 'Child behaviour problems and parental attitudes.' *Child Develop.*, **32**, 51.

PIDGEON, D. A. (1960) 'A national survey of the ability and attainment of children at three age levels.' *Brit. J. educ. Psychol.*, **30**, 124.

PILZER, E. (1952) 'Disturbed children who make good school adjustment.' *Smith Coll. Stud. Soc. Wk.*, **22**, 193.

POWERS, E., and WITMER, H. L. (1951) *An experiment in the prevention of delinquency.* New York: Columbia University Press.

PRESTON, G. H., and SHEPLER, W. MCL. (1930) 'A study of problems of "normal" children.' *Amer. J. Orthopsychiat.*, **1**, 245.

PRINGLE, M. L. K., BUTLER, N. R., and DAVIE, R. (1966) *11000 Seven-year-olds.* London: Longmans.

REXFORD, E. N., and SCHLEIFER, M. (1956) 'A follow-up of a psychiatric study of 57 antisocial young children.' *Ment. Hyg.*, **40**, 196.

REYNOLDS, M. M. (1928) 'Negativism in pre-school children.' Contribution to *Education*, No. 28, New York Teachers College, Columbia University.

RITHOLZ, S. (1959) *Children's behaviour*. New York: Bookmen Associates.

ROBINS, L. N. (1970) 'Follow-up studies of behaviour disorders in children.' In HARE, E. H., and WING, J. K. (eds.) *Psychiatric epidemiology*. Nuffield Provincial Hospitals Trusts.

ROBINSON, B. H. (1951) In Child Guidance Inter-clinic Conference, *9th Follow-up on child guidance cases*. London: National Association for Mental Health.

RODRIGUES, A., RODRIGUES, M., and EISENBERG, L. (1959) 'The outcome of school phobia: a follow-up study based on 41 cases.' *Amer. J. Psychiat.*, **116**, 540.

ROGERS, C. R. (1942) 'Mental health findings in three elementary schools.' *Educ. Res. Bull.*, (Ohio State University), **21**(3), 69.

RUTTER, M., BIRCH, H. G., THOMAS, A., and CHESS, S. (1964) 'Temperamental characteristics in infancy and the later development of behaviour disorders.' *Brit. J. Psychiat.*, **110**, 651.

RUTTER, M., and GRAHAM, P. (1966) 'Psychiatric disorders in 10- and 11-year-old children.' *Proc. Roy. Soc. Med.* **59**, 382.

RUTTER, M., TIZARD, J. and WHITMORE, K. (eds.) (1970) *Education, Health and Behaviour*. London: Longmans.

RYLE, A. (1963) 'Psychotherapy by the non-psychiatrist.' *Proc. Roy. Soc. Med.*, **56**, 834.

SCHONELL, F. J. (1952) 'The development of educational research in Great Britain: 7 Maladjusted children.' *Brit. J. educ. Psychol.*, **22**, 30.

SCHRUPP, M. H., and GJERDE, C. M. (1953) 'Teacher growth in attitudes toward behaviour problems of children.' *J. educ. Psychol.*, **44**, 203.

SCOTT, W. A. (1958a) 'Research definitions of mental health and mental illness.' *Psychol. Bull.*, **55**, 29.

SCOTT, W. A. (1958b) 'Social psychological correlates of mental illness and mental health.' *Psychol. Bull.*, **55**, 65.

SHEPHERD, M., and COOPER, B. (1964) 'Epidemiology and mental disorder: a review.' *J. Neurol. Neurosurg. Psychiat.*, **27**, 277.

SPENCE, J., WALTON, W., MILLER, F. J. W., and COURT, S. D. M. (1954) *A thousand families in Newcastle upon Tyne*. London: Oxford University Press.

STEIN, Z. A., and SUSSER, M. (1967) 'The social dimensions of a symptom: a socio-medical study of enuresis.' *Soc. Sci. and Med.*, **1**, 183.

STOTT, D. H. (1958) *The social adjustment of children: manual to the Bristol Social Adjustment Guides*. London: University of London Press.

SULLY, J. (1892) *The human mind: a textbook of psychology*. London: Longmans.

TAYLOR, T. C. (1968) Unpublished information.

TERMAN, L. M. (ed.) (1925) *Genetic studies of genius: Vol. I. Physical traits of 1000 gifted children*. Stanford University Press.

THOMPSON, C. E. (1940) 'The attitudes of various groups toward behaviour problems of children.' *J. abnorm. soc. Psychol.*, **35**, 120.

TIMMS, N. W. (1968) 'Child guidance service: a pilot study.' In MCLACHLAN, G. (ed.) *Problems and progress in medical care*. London: Oxford University Press.

TRAISMAN, A. S., and TRAISMAN, H. S. (1958) 'Thumb and finger-sucking: a study of 2650 infants and children.' *J. Pediat.*, **52**, 566.

TREVELYAN, G. M. (1942) *English social history*. London: Longmans.

TYERMAN, M. J. (1968) *Truancy*. London: University of London Press.

ULLMAN, C. A. (1952) *Identification of maladjusted school children*. Public Health Monogr. (Washington), 7.

VALENTINE, C. W. (1956) *The normal child*. Pelican. Harmondsworth, Middlesex: Penguin Books.

VAN LAAR, F., RUSBACH, H. W., and DE HAAS, J. H. (1962) 'Menstruatiestoornissen bij schoolgaands adolescenten.' *Tijdschr. soc. Geneesk.*, **40**, 44.

VON HARNACK, G.-A. (1953) 'Wesen und soziale Bedingtheit frühkindlicher Verhaltensstörungen.' *Bibl. Paediat.*, Fasc. 55.

VON HARNACK, G.-A. (1958) *Nervose Verhaltensstörungen beim Schulkind*. Stuttgart: Georg Thieme Verlag.

WALBY, J. H., and MacLOUGHLIN, A. L. (1963) 'Health and the 11 Plus Examination.' *Med. Offr.*, **109**, 137.

WALLACE, R. (1935) 'A study of the relationship between emotional tone of the home and adjustment status in cases referred to a travelling child guidance clinic.' *J. Juvenile Res.*, **19**, 205.

WECHSLER, D. (1931) 'The incidence and significance of finger-nail biting in children.' *Psychoanal. Rev.*, **18**, 201.

WHITING, J. W. M., and CHILD, I. L. (1953) *Child training and personality: a cross-cultural study*. New Haven: Yale University Press.

WICKMAN, E. K. (1928) *Children's behaviour and teachers' attitudes*. New York: Commonwealth Fund.

WILE, I. S., NEARY, L., NOVOGRAD, L., MACE, L., and DAVIS, R. (1934) 'The continuity of the neurotic processes.' *Amer. J. Orthopsychiat.*, **4**, 49.

WISENTHAL, M. (1965) 'Sex differences in attitudes and attainment in junior schools.' *Brit. J. educ. Psychol.*, **35**, 79.

WITMER, H. L. (1933a) 'The outcome of treatment in a child guidance clinic.' *Smith Coll. Stud. soc. Wk.*, **3**, 341.

WITMER, H. L. (1933b) 'Parental behaviour as an index to the probable outcome of treatment in a child guidance clinic.' *Amer. J. Orthopsychiat.*, **3**, 431.

WITMER, H. L. (1935) 'A comparison of treatment results in various types of child guidance clinics.' *Amer. J. Orthopsychiat.*, **5**, 351.

WITMER, H. L. (1940) *Psychiatric clinics for children.* New York: Commonwealth Fund.

WOLFF, S. (1961) 'Symptomatology and outcome of pre-school children with behaviour disorders attending a child guidance clinic.' *J. Child Psychol. Psychiat.*, **2**, 269.

WOLFF, S. (1967) 'Behavioural characteristics of primary school children referred to a psychiatric department.' *Brit. J. Psychiat.*, **113**, 885.

YARROW, L. J. (1961) 'Maternal deprivation: towards an empirical and conceptual re-evaluation.' *Psychol. Bull.*, **58**, 459.

YOUNG-MASTEN, I. (1938) 'Behaviour problems of elementary school children: a descriptive and comparative study.' *Genet. Psychol. Monogr.*, **20**(2), 123.

YOURMAN, J. (1932) 'Children identified by their teachers as problems.' *J. educ. Psychol.*, **6**, 334.

Author index

Subject index

References to figures are in italics